Waking Up
from MS

Waking Up from MS

MY JOURNEY TO HEALTH, HEALING, AND LIVING SYMPTOM FREE

* * *

Kellie Alderton

ISBN: 0692771824
ISBN 13: 9780692771822

This book is dedicated to my greatest loves, Sarah and Gregory. Follow your dreams relentlessly, have faith, and your true purpose will reveal itself.

Contents

Acknowledgments

I WANT TO THANK MY mom for her love, loyalty, friendship, compassion, and strength. You have taught me so much about life. Thank you for always supporting me in every single interest I've had through the years and encouraging me to follow my dreams. You've been with me every step of the way while writing this book, and that means the world to me. I aspire to be like you each and every day. I love you more!

To my true love, best friend, and soul mate—my husband, Greg. Thank you for always believing in me and supporting me in every way on this journey of healing and finding my life's purpose.

Kim thanks for always being here for me. I hope you can continue to use this book as a stepping stone for your complete healing.

I am forever grateful to my friend and colleague Greg M. Thank you for pointing me down the right path—the path that saved my life. Words cannot express my appreciation and gratitude to you!

Jodi, thank you for bringing me the opportunity that changed my life forever! Thanks for all the help you've given me with *MS Free for ALL*.

Denise, thank you for editing my author photo and your creative insight, vision, and encouragement while trying to figure out the cover photo.

My BFF, Tammy, I appreciate everything we've been through personally and professionally—so many great memories! You've taught me that you can have it all and still have fun in the process. Thanks for being a great sounding board throughout this process and encouraging me in everything I do. (atiakow)

Paul, thanks for your friendship and support in everything I do.

Mayra, I am grateful that we started this book-writing journey together—what an adventure. Thank you for always believing in me and encouraging me to get my vision out into the world.

Antonio, thank you for your continued friendship and encouragement, especially while I wrote this.

Jan Fraser, thank you for opening your home to me and Mayra for our writers' retreat and for teaching me this process. Thanks for instilling confidence in me that I could write this.

I have to thank Jack Canfield. Your Breakthrough to Success Training was a pivotal point in my life. You taught me to take 100 percent responsibility for my goals and my life. The tools I learned from you not only helped me with this book, but also helped me transform my life with MS.

Debbie H., I am so truly blessed that we met at that MS-support-group meeting. You have been such a wonderful friend and confidant. I'm very excited to be a part of your own journey to beating MS.

Jennifer and Sharon, your friendship, strength, and faith have helped me see things in the right way, with the right perspective. Thank you for your constant encouragement and love.

Judie, you're a great friend. Thanks for your continued encouragement throughout this book-writing process.

Alice, thank you for being such a great supporter and sounding board while I've been working on this project.

Dr. Donsbach, thank you for opening my eyes to the possibility of healing and beating MS.

Dr. Kelly Geritano, you were the first stop on my road to healing. Thank you for taking care of me and my family during these past fifteen years. Your knowledge and support mean so much.

Dr. Marie Tholl-Pappas, thank you for giving such great care to me and my family.

Tina Forshey, thank you for the beautiful picture and sharing your creative ideas with me for the cover.

Ayden and Danny, thanks for helping me through trial and errors with the cover. That was fun. Love you both so much!

Bill C., thank you for believing in me and encouraging me to keep moving forward in helping people with MS.

My Vollara family, I am so blessed to be a part of this company whose products have helped pave the way to my healing. The leadership and friendships I have found here have been such a blessing to me and my entire family.

To all my family and friends who have supported and encouraged me on this journey, I am forever grateful. I love you all!

To my MS family, your courage, strength, and determination to beat MS have forever inspired me. Never give up!

Preface

My husband, Greg, and I walked out of the support-group meeting and I began sobbing. I looked at him and said, "I need to help these people; it doesn't have to be this way." We had just been listening to a doctor describe the worst possible information on MS, saying there was no cure, and that drug therapy was the only way to extend our lives a few more years. I saw a room full of people who were eager for answers, now deflated and hopeless. I thought to myself, *How can I tell them I was in their shoes before? How can I tell them not to give up? How can I tell them there is another way? How can I give them hope?* That's where this book's journey began.

Fear, ignorance, and lack of knowledge had kept me on the MS medical treadmill. I kept running and following the protocols, not knowing there was any other way to live with this disease. And let me tell you, it was exhausting.

As many of you also living with MS may understand, for years and years, I was walking through life with this disease, simply waiting for the next flare-up to take over my life.

Why was I waiting for the next flare-up? Because my doctors said that's all we could do.

Not a day goes by that I don't feel for people with multiple sclerosis—my MS family, not because they have MS but because most people get the diagnosis and think it's a death sentence. They don't realize they have options, they don't realize they have choices, and they definitely don't realize they can live healthy, happy, and productive lives.

I guess the easiest thing to do is go back to the beginning, back to 1988. That's when I started on this journey with MS. At the ripe old age of seventeen I was diagnosed with relapsing-remitting multiple sclerosis, and the first thing my doctor said was, "There is no cure." I heard my family whispering, telling everyone about my diagnosis, but being young, naïve, and not having a clue what multiple sclerosis was, I just figured it would all work out. You know teenagers; we think we're indestructible!

At seventeen, I was walking around with a black eye patch, since I had just been diagnosed with not only multiple sclerosis, but also optic neuritis. I was the laughingstock of my high school. (You know how everyone likes to be different there.)

I had no idea what was going on with my body; it just wasn't working right. It was as if something else was controlling it. When I finally took the time to find out some info on MS, I learned that this disease was very different, very debilitating, very frustrating, and terribly scary for a kid. I thought I could possibly die. The people with MS who I saw in pictures looked scary and bleak. While in high school, I was so exhausted that I was bedridden for weeks at a time. Often I thought there was no hope, no treatment, no cure, and definitely no future for me!

I went through years and years of trials and tribulations, as I'm sure many of you who have multiple sclerosis understand. I've had many challenges during these twenty-nine years of living with this disease—depression;

panic attacks; desperation; chronic fatigue; optic neuritis; tremendous aches and pains; Bell's palsy; numbness and tingling; brain fog; loss of function in my hands, arms, and legs; and drop foot. I've had weird eye problems that some of my doctors have never experienced with their other MS patients, and frankly, they just didn't know what to do with me. This was my MS life, and I just kept going day by day, year by year, waiting for the next flare-up to happen. Living like that was a mess, and at times in the beginning of this journey, I was full of fear!

Now, let's move forward to 1995. I was twenty-four years old, and I felt healthy and strong throughout my very first pregnancy. I thought I had beaten this disease, until a few months after my daughter Sarah's birth, when she almost slipped out of my hands because I couldn't feel her in my arms. That was really scary! And it was a reminder to me that MS was always lurking in the background, waiting to come back and disrupt my life.

This is a brief version of some of the issues I've had while living with multiple sclerosis for the past twenty-nine years. I'm doing this intentionally because I don't want to focus on the flare-ups, the exacerbations, the struggles, and the *fear* that I know anyone with multiple sclerosis will undoubtedly understand. I don't want you to focus on them either. I want you to focus on repair, healing, inspiration, and figuring out ways to be healthy. That's why I wrote this book. I want this to be a story of triumphs, new beginnings, and new ideas that perhaps you have never thought about or known about. The number-one thing I want this book to do is bring you hope!

In 1988, I thought having MS was a life sentence—a life that could never be truly enjoyed or fulfilled. I'm here to tell you it doesn't have to be that way. I am living proof of how to overcome multiple sclerosis. I hope this book will help you on your journey to waking up from MS!

The Awakening Begins

In 2001, I felt that MS was draining me little by little, day by day. I was taking two to three naps a day. MS was wreaking havoc on my mind and body, and it was definitely killing my spirit. This disease was so sporadic, reckless, debilitating, and utterly unpredictable. I was told over and over that there was no cure. Still, I prayed that somehow things would get better.

One of the troubling things about MS is that people cannot understand the struggle its victims are going through on a daily basis. I could go hang out with family or friends, and to them I looked normal. Everything was happening on the inside; people couldn't see my fatigue, couldn't feel my aches and pains, and couldn't understand my brain fog. That was another point in this journey when I really understood how much of an invisible disease this can be at times for its sufferers.

In 2001, one of the most significant and life-changing events happened to me. My sister-in-law Jodi introduced me and my husband to a new business opportunity at Ecoquest, which is now Vollara International. The company focuses on green technologies, whole-food supplements, and healthy living—many topics I was clueless about.

When I joined that company, I was introduced to many health-conscious people who knew how to live right, eat right, *and* think right to be healthy. In that company, a colleague gave me information that *rocked my world*!

Yes, it was that profound.

I heard about healing, repair, and vitality—information I had never heard before from anyone involved in treating my MS. I was told that there are other ways to deal with MS.

I learned the following information:

* MS could be a vitamin deficiency.
* I could be healthy.
* I could have a wonderful quality of life.
* I could have a long life.

That information shook me to my core; I was in total disbelief and, of course, very skeptical. At first, I was thinking to myself, *My doctors never, ever told me this*. And I had been working with these doctors for more than a decade.

I took some time and thought about this information, and I thought, *Hey, I'll try this new course*. And that information literally *saved my life*.

That day in 2001 was when I started to change my life, change my ideas, and change my thinking. I had always felt there had to be something more for me and my life than letting this disease control it, and at that point, I knew there was; I was on a different path.

I was told repeatedly by my doctors that there was no hope, no true way of healing, and definitely no cure, so I was now embarking into uncharted territory on a quest to figure out this disease and figure out how to heal my body. And most importantly, I wanted to know why this information isn't readily given to all MS patients.

This story chronicles some of my journey with multiple sclerosis. It has real information about what I've done and also what others are doing to help their MS. It has information about healthy living and new ways of thinking. After all, I believe this journey is about sharing information and tips that have worked—but more importantly, I want to inspire you to want more for yourself and your life with MS.

I've always looked at MS as just a thing. It has never defined me, and I have never wanted it to define how I live my life. I have learned some key strategies and information about beating this disease, and I have a wonderful quality of life, feeling healthy, strong, and grateful.

Here is what I hope you will learn in this book:

- What I did to combat the chronic fatigue
- What I did to combat the brain fog
- What I did to transform my body
- What I did to transform my mind
- What I did to transform my heart
- What I did to become symptom-free
- What we can do each and every day to lead healthy lives

God willing, this is what I want for everyone suffering from MS. I think we can do this one person at a time, one story at a time, and one helping hand at a time. This book is straight from my heart. I want to give each person who reads it hope! I want to give each person who reads this a stepping stone of new ideas and different ways of thinking, in the hopes of turning their own disease around.

I have invested many years into education, research, and investigation on this subject. This information was compiled to inspire you, motivate you, and perhaps help you change your whole perspective about this disease. At the end of the day, I know I am healthy, I am strong, and I have overcome my MS because of God's grace and mercy. I believe I must now do my part by speaking out and offering a helping hand to others. I want to give you a vision of a future where multiple sclerosis does not rule your life.

CHAPTER 1
My Story

"While we may not be able to control all that happens
to us, we can control what happens inside us."

—*Ben Franklin*

In 1988, I was a normal seventeen-year-old, a senior in high school. It was almost spring, and I was glad winter was over. I was always active in sports; I loved basketball and especially softball. My graduation was only a few months away. I was really excited about my future and all that life after high school would offer me.

Thinking back across all those years, I try to pinpoint exactly when I started having health issues. I think it all began in the months of February and March, when I was starting to experience some odd things. I was under a lot of stress from typical high school issues—friends, my boyfriend, family, and exams. I was so tired that for a few weeks, all I could do was sleep. I remember telling my mom, "I'm just so exhausted; I can't go to school."

You can imagine how parents feel when their kids say they are sick for two weeks straight and are just lying around, doing nothing. They thought I was faking. I went to the doctor, and he thought it was just a virus. He didn't give me any meds; he just said to get plenty of rest and drink lots of fluids. For some reason, I didn't have the energy to do anything. It was very odd.

After a few days, I began feeling like my old self again, and I went back to the daily grind of high-school life.

As the end of April came around, I was gearing up for my new season of softball. I had been a part of this league since I was seven. I made the all-star team ten years in a row. I really enjoyed the game, my team, the friends I made throughout the league, and the competition. Driving to the first day of practice, I noticed that my eyes weren't right. It seemed like there was a horrible glare on the window. The sun was starting to go down a bit, so I didn't give it another thought.

After arriving at the softball field, I put my cleats on, and I was excited to see my old friends. The coach announced to the team, "Go anywhere, and take a position; I'm going to hit around for warm-ups." I thought, *Cool, I'll start in center field*—an easy position for someone who's been playing as long as I had been. I figured I'd start in the outfield, move to the infield, and then go bat. The coach started hitting around, and it was softball as usual. We were all excited to be getting back into the swing of things.

Standing in center field, I eagerly awaited the ball. Then, all of a sudden, whack—a perfect fly ball to center field, a perfect hit to me. I started running in to catch it, and *wow*, I couldn't believe it; it flew right over my head. I totally misjudged it, which was odd for me. I had played softball for so many years that I was easily accustomed to waiting out the ball coming at me, and I knew where you had to be to catch it. *Hmm*, I thought, *this is really weird.*

Coach called out, "Let's try that again, Kellie!" So again, there was a whack, and another perfect fly ball came at me; I was even in perfect alignment with it. I brought up my arms to catch it, but I was too late. It hit me right in the face. Ouch! That really hurt!

I don't know what hurt more, my face or my pride. I started laughing; I couldn't believe it. This was so out of character for me and especially out of character for someone who'd been playing for a decade. I sat in the field for a minute, trying to understand what had just happened, when the coach called me in to bat. He asked whether everything was OK out there. I said, "Yeah. I'm not sure what's going on."

He said, "Are you ready to take some hits?" Of course I was ready; I would do anything to get out of this embarrassing situation. It was the first practice back, and I was a mess. I had to redeem myself.

I grabbed a bat and started taking some practice swings. It seemed like old times, comfortable and easy. I stepped up to the plate, dug in with my back foot, brought my elbows up in perfect form, and got ready to clobber the ball. The pitcher threw me a beautiful pitch. I took what I thought was an awesome swing, and I missed. Not only did I miss, I spun around what seemed like a million times. I felt like a five-year-old, a novice, just learning to hit the ball for the first time. I could not believe it! I was very unstable and shaky; I didn't know what was happening. I just laughed and called to the pitcher, "This is nuts. Let's go! Pitch again. That's only strike one." I was laughing cautiously.

I got set. I took a full swing around, missing the ball again and making yet another strike. I was so angry and confused and didn't understand what was going on. The bat felt heavier with each swing. I was totally misjudging the pitch, my swing—everything. *OK*, I thought, *one more try*. Again, one more strike. No way. This did not just happen. No one strikes out in sixteen-inch softball. My coach benched me. He was just as frustrated as I was. He came over and asked whether I was trying to fail, whether I wanted to be on this team. I said, "Are you kidding? I have no idea what's going on." He told me to go home and come back to the next practice. Our games and practices went from April to August. We played for all those months and all those years under high-voltage power lines. No one thought anything about it at the time, but I have always wondered if that was a catalyst in my getting MS. I thought this was very interesting, as my twin sister and I were both exposed to that same environmental factor; she played softball all those years too. My sister was diagnosed at the age of eighteen with RRMS (relapsing remitting multiple sclerosis). I also have another friend who played softball with us at those same fields year after year; she has also been diagnosed with MS. Was that a contributing factor?

While driving home from that first practice, I felt confused, frustrated, and embarrassed. I was in my parents' brand-new car, and I had to keep closing one eye to see properly. I even hit the curb a few times when making turns. I couldn't judge how far away objects were; it was really strange. When I got home, I told my mom and dad that there was something wrong with my eyes. My dad said, "No, there's not. You probably just need new glasses."

I said, "I don't think so; something is not right. I can't see."

He responded as most dads would: "You'll be fine." He was, I'm sure, thinking I was overreacting.

The next day, I went to my boyfriend's house. His mom handed me a stack of family pictures to look at, and I couldn't grab them from her. She held them out, and I was either reaching too high or too low. We just laughed, and she put them in my hand to review. I was also having problems in class, seeing papers and the chalkboard, and it was even difficult to see down the hallways of the school. I thought maybe Dad was right; maybe I *did* need new glasses.

A few days later, my mom took me to the eye doctor for what we were thinking would be a new prescription.

At the doctor's office, he gave me some tests, and he seemed very quiet. He abruptly stopped and had me leave the room. He proceeded to tell my mom that I needed to go to a neurologist and that I needed to go right away. Talk about scary; I wasn't even sure what a neurologist was.

The next morning, I had an appointment with a pediatric neurologist. To me, there was a bright spot: I was excited about having a day off from school. I was thinking, *Long weekend for me.* I figured I'd be fine. I had no idea what was going to happen next.

When I arrived at the neurologist's office, he conducted what I now understand to be the typical testing for MS: follow the doctor's finger without moving your head. Unfortunately, however, I could not keep my head still. It had to follow my eyes. I kept apologizing. I told him, "Really, I'm not a difficult patient. I'm trying." And I laughed. He had me squeeze his fingers, to test my strength. He had me stand with my eyes closed, arms out on the sides, and I was swaying all over. I couldn't take my finger and reach around to touch my nose, I kept missing. He hit all my joints with his little mallet (fun stuff). I even had to read some numbers out of a little black book for depth perception. Guess what? I had none.

He said we needed to get an MRI right away. I didn't have a clue what an MRI was. He explained, "It's just a more detailed X-ray of your head." When I arrived at the MRI center, it was a bit scary. I had never seen such a contraption. You lie down on a table, and you get pushed into a large tube. It felt like I was in a coffin—small, confining, and cold—and the loud noises that came out of the machine were freaking me out. Remember, this was way back in 1988. The MRI was a lot different back then compared to what we have now.

Next, everything was quick, quick, quick. We had the results right away. I learned I had multiple sclerosis. I had more than twenty lesions on my brain. *Hmm*, I thought, *multiple sclerosis.* That didn't even register with me. I had no idea what it was, and I'm sure no one in my family did either.

Multiple sclerosis was not well known or even talked about much back in the '80s, and, of course, in those days, we didn't have Google, Pubmed, or WebMD to help find information. My official diagnosis was relapsing remitting multiple sclerosis. Approximately 85 percent of people with MS are initially diagnosed with RRMS (NationalMSSociety.org).

I had optic neuritis (blurred or double vision), dizziness, loss of balance, pain and numbness in my limbs, and extreme fatigue. I went home with the diagnosis and some meds from the doctor to try to help my dizziness. He handed my mom a few brochures, and we were off. There was definite confusion in my household, and I overheard many whispered phone calls from my parents to other family members. All we could do was keep going and deal with my condition and information as it became available.

A few weeks after my diagnosis, my eye was still bad, but at that point, I knew that I had missed too much school already. I had to get back and get ready for finals. After all, I was a senior, and those were my last steps so I could graduate.

The doctor recommended I wear an eye patch to help stabilize me. I said, "What? You know I'm seventeen; I can't possibly wear that thing!" Talk about standing out like a sore thumb. Being a teenager and looking like a pirate was not going to be too cool. That seemed like the worst thing that could happen to me—forget the diagnosis of MS, but an eyepatch? What was this guy trying to do to me?

I did finally obey the doctor's order. (The patch actually helped; when I took the patch off, I became very dizzy and disoriented from the optic neuritis.) Yes, a few people made fun of me, and probably a lot more were mean behind my back. You know, kids loved making pirate comments to me. I did my best to try to make a lovely fashion statement out of my eye patch. I don't think it worked very well.

MS was new to me and my family, and it was really not talked about in the medical community at that time. When I got back to school, and people learned that I had multiple sclerosis, a few students ran up to me and apologized. They asked me whether I would end up like the rest of Jerry's kids. Yes, Jerry's kids!

For those of you who don't know Jerry Lewis, he's hosted some of the biggest telethons for muscular dystrophy. They introduced kids in wheelchairs, and you could see how much they were suffering. They became known as Jerry's kids. Well, muscular dystrophy is not multiple sclerosis. In the beginning, I was very confused; I didn't know what the heck I had. I thought I could be like one of Jerry's kids in a wheelchair. It really freaked me out.

After I had missed several weeks of school, the deans and most faculty members I ran into knew I had been diagnosed with multiple sclerosis. They all said "I'm sorry"; they hugged me and offered me help and encouragement so I could get through the last few weeks of school. Several teachers felt bad for me, I guess, and waived my final exams. I cautiously said thanks.

The reactions of several of my teachers even became alarming. I'll never forget my home economics teacher's reaction—when I saw her, she cried. This teacher was very disciplined and strict. She reminded me of a stern Julia Childs; my teacher never cracked a smile and was never very personable with any of us, so her reaction made me think I was going to die. I was grateful for the passing grades I received for some of my finals and for the kind sentiments, but I was still shaken by the extreme reactions.

I felt like I was in the Twilight Zone—like I was having an out-of-body experience. I was feeling every single ache and pain MS had to offer. Yes, I had the eye patch, but no one could see what was really going on inside me. This was the first time I realized this was a very personal and internal disease.

This was one of many, many experiences and challenges for me as I learned to live with multiple sclerosis under the normal medical protocols for the next thirteen years.

I really didn't understand this disease for many years. I was a young kid, and quite frankly, MS scared me if I thought about it too much. No one in my family really talked about it. I didn't investigate anything about MS—its signs or symptoms. I was afraid of what was next and what I could be facing right around the corner, going from doctor to doctor to try to help me. Throughout my illness, I have been in hospitals in Germany, Colorado, and Illinois, dealing with my disease and my symptoms.

My everyday issues, as for many MS sufferers, were fatigue, migraines, depression, anxiety, aches and pains, numbness and tingling, optic neuritis, Bell's palsy, as well as many challenges with my limbs. Sometimes one whole side of my body would be numb and hard to move. Other times, I just had problems with my hands, arms, or feet. On several occasions, the doctors weren't really sure how to treat me other than with steroids, since that was the standard protocol back then.

Since I was so out of touch with this disease in the beginning and what it could do to me, I felt like the more I ignored it, the better off I would be. I had no idea that there were options for me to be proactive about dealing with this disease. I had no idea of the causes of MS or what things I may have actually been doing to make it worse. I didn't know there may be environmental factors that could not only cause it, but also cause an exacerbation. I didn't know about the studies on how to heal, how to eat, or how to exercise. I guess the whole theory that you don't know what you don't know applies here.

This was the period I call BA or "before alternatives"—the alternatives that I believed saved me.

At a couple of points in my life, I had to stop working, as my employers would not allow me to take time off while having a flare-up. I still wanted to be productive and do something for my family. I wanted to do something to keep active and not just lie around the house, waiting for MS to rule my life.

That's when my sister-in-law Jodi introduced me and my husband to the work-from-home business Ecoquest, which is now known as Vollara International. This company is amazing, and focuses on healthy living, healthy products, healthy technologies, and definitely healthy, success-minded thinking. That allowed me the opportunity to be at home with no worries about what was happening with my disease. It also gave me the opportunity to help others so I didn't focus on my own illness all day. Have you ever noticed how easy it is to get so sidetracked and become laser focused on our own health challenges so that everything seems overwhelming, out of control, and dismal? That was exactly how I felt at times.

This new opportunity really changed everything for me, and I believe it was the catalyst in my becoming healthier, for several reasons. First, I was introduced to the idea of supplementation and how important it is, even if I didn't have the best diet at the time. I learned that if my body was out of sync nutritionally, it could lead to a host of health crises, not just MS. Secondly, I was working in an environment focused on healthy living, which changed how I live my everyday life, from what I eat, to the air I breathe, to the water I drink, to the way I washed my laundry—(yes, there is a completely healthy and environmentally friendly way to do that)—and most importantly, the attitude I have and my overall expectations in life. This was such a breath of fresh air for me. Every day I learned something new, not only to help my health, but also to help my family; 2017 is my sixteenth year in my health-focused business, and I am blessed that this opportunity crossed my path. I think about what would have been if I was never given this opportunity, this information, and these knowledgeable friends to help me on this journey to improved health. I wonder how bad I would be today. This is the reason I am sharing my story with you. I want this book to be thought-provoking; I hope to bring you knowledge, understanding, and choices!

My Identical Twin

As I stated earlier, I am an identical twin. Studies suggest that MS is found more often in twins. My twin sister, Kim, has been more debilitated with MS than I. Kim was actually exhibiting symptoms of MS two years before I did, at the age of fifteen. She had drop foot and was put in a partial cast and on steroids. The doctors didn't tell us back then that problems like drop foot and problems with limbs were something very much associated with multiple sclerosis. Kim was diagnosed at the age of eighteen with relapsing remitting MS, a year after me. Even when I was diagnosed, we did not correlate her past health issues with her having MS.

I know the school of thought is that multiple sclerosis is hereditary. Kim and I have had very active MS with consistent flare-ups throughout the years, but is it really hereditary? Is it found more often in twins merely because of the sibling relationship? I wondered whether it was because we were both exposed to the same factors—we ate the same diet, drank the same things, and were both exposed to the same environmental toxins. Kim played softball right there next to me for all those years under those power lines, we cooked the same foods year in and year out in the microwave and that makes me wonder.

What's interesting about my sister is that she had gone the traditional medical route the whole time while dealing with her MS, and she has had consistent challenges and flare-ups for years.

Why, you might ask, has Kim not done exactly what I have done to become healthier and stronger? Well, that's a great question and one I get asked quite frequently. The easy answer is that Kim is at a different place than I am as far as alternative treatments. Kim is like many MS sufferers who've had the disease for any length of time: that's what they're used to. The daily ins and outs of MS become acceptable. I don't think it's intentional; it's just something that happens. My sister does not live the life I live. Some personal issues cause her tremendous stress every day. She also deals with stress differently than I do. Even though we are in the same family, she has a different support system around her. I do work with Kim consistently to try to help her go another way, and thankfully, step by step, she is making changes and making progress. The good news is that she stopped all DMDs (disease-modifying drugs). You'll find that I'm not an advocate of them, and I'll explain more later in the book. Kim has recently started looking at alternatives too. Now the key point in her becoming healthier will be to change her diet, add more supplements, and also do plenty of rehabilitation therapy to reverse the effects that MS has had on her body, specifically in her legs. When you are living with MS for any length of time and you become debilitated and lack exercise, you can have muscle atrophy; that's where Kim's legs are at this point. I am hopeful that she will have a complete turnaround in the coming months and years.

The Long MS Walk

I like to think that those of us who have MS are a family, an MS community. We're all in this together. In most cases, that's exactly how it is and how I've been received. I've made many friends via social networking, support groups, and MS functions. I want to share this story because this experience was a real eye-opener to me about how others, even if they have multiple sclerosis, may perceive people or situations.

In 1999, I registered for and participated in a local MS walk. It was fantastic. I was thrilled to be able to walk, especially because two weeks prior, I just had been released from the hospital, where I was being treated for drop foot. I was having a lot of pain, and my body was very unstable. After five days of therapy in the hospital, I was good to go, feeling great, walking normally, and ready to take on the world.

This MS walk had special meaning for me, considering the state I had been in just a few weeks prior. This would be the first function that my awesome, soon-to-be-husband, Greg, was involved in. The walk was extremely exciting for me, just because I could fully participate. As we were crossing the finish line, I felt so happy and yet somber, as many of my fellow MS sufferers could not walk. They had family members walking for them.

I started talking with some ladies who also had MS. They were in wheelchairs. I was happy to speak with them until one of the ladies said to me very sternly, "You don't have MS!"

Taken aback, I said, "Excuse me?"

She said angrily, "There's no way you have MS."

I said, "I'm sorry. Do I know you?"

She said, "No."

I took a deep breath, trying to get my wits about me. I began to tell her a little about myself—when I was diagnosed, what my symptoms were, what my testing was like, and I shared that I had been released from the hospital just a few weeks prior because of an exacerbation. She seemed pretty angry with me. I had no clue what I had done to offend this woman. It was very odd. Was she angry at me because I was doing so well? Was she angry at me because I was laughing, having fun, and talking with everyone? To this day, I'm not sure why she was angry.

I've also come across people through business associations who don't have MS. I've told them my story, and how I healed. They said there's no way I beat my MS through diet, nutrition, green products, and alternative therapies. That *used* to be upsetting to me, but through lots of growth and personal development, I understand that what people think of me is really none of my business. My true friends and family know what I've been through, and they have always been supportive. Others have their own issues, and I guess it makes them feel better to try and tear others down. This is why we must always understand that we cannot presume to know what others have gone through in their lives. Until you walk in their shoes, it's really better to keep your opinion to yourself.

The point of these personal experiences is to let you know that you may not only have negative feedback from family, friends or business colleagues; it can also come from fellow MS sufferers. I try not to take it to heart. I've learned that when some people are hurting, they tend to want to hurt others too. Also, if you are the one who is angry or very negative, it's time to take a look at ways you can turn that around. It will be better for your overall health. I will give you steps and techniques in the book about how you can do that.

I feel that all of us living with MS should stand by each other. We're all in this fight together!

STAYING-ACTIVE PHILOSOPHY

Another important factor to my overall health is that I strive to stay active. You'll see a lot of information throughout the book about staying active, and you can start simple steps right away to help your MS. I like to go out with my friends and family. I love to dance. I love to travel. I love to be around people. I love to go out to eat. I love speaking publicly, where I can encourage and motivate others. I love to exercise—I like to participate in Pilates and weightlifting as part of my regimen—and I will talk about that in more detail later in the book.

My philosophy of staying active not only means physically; you must stay active mentally too. I enjoy being a lifetime learner. I love to learn as much as I can about many topics. I've focused on healthy, positive-minded people like Jack Canfield, Tony Robbins, Dani Johnson, Robin Sharma, John Maxwell, Max Lucado, Jim Bunch, Brian Tracy, Napoleon Hill, Dale Carnegie, Dr. Wayne Dyer, Maxwell Maltz, Lee Strobel, and Louise Hay. I've studied and learned about holistic nutrition, juicing, different diets, healthy living, and alternative therapies, and I've definitely found tons of information on multiple sclerosis. Information and resources are changing daily, and I am always open to learning more so I can stay healthy and help others.

What you will see in this book is real information that has led me to an evolution of thinking, succeeding, and overcoming MS. I hope I can help inspire and challenge you to become your best health advocate and meet your MS head on.

My heart goes out to all MS sufferers, their loved ones, and those who care for them. I know the struggles are difficult; there are ups and downs, many trials and tribulations. We must be strong in order to overcome this disease. My hope is to unite the MS community in an attempt to share knowledge and ideas and to help others on their journeys to waking up from MS!

I am not a physician. You should always follow the advice of your trusted health-care professional. I am sharing my personal experiences with you. This should not be a substitute for medical advice.

CHAPTER 2

What Is MS?

"Sometimes the diagnosis is worse than the disease!"

—*Unknown*

MS, or multiple sclerosis, is a disease that affects the brain and spinal cord, resulting in loss of vision, balance, coordination, and muscle control. It can even cause sensations such as numbness, tingling, or feelings of heaviness in the limbs. With MS, the immune system actually damages the nerves of the brain and spinal cord.

MS gets its name from the buildup of scar tissue (sclerosis) in the brain and spinal cord. The scar tissue, or plaque, forms when the protective and insulating myelin covering the nerves is destroyed. (In an MRI of the brain, these plaques look similar to cavities on your teeth that you can see in a dental X-ray.) This is a process called demyelination. Without the myelin, signals transmitted throughout the brain and spinal cord are disrupted. It is this breakdown that causes the MS symptoms, and the body literally attacks itself.

MS is two to three times more common in females than in males, and its occurrence is unusual before adolescence (although it is happening to younger children now more frequently). I know a lot of people who've been diagnosed with MS in their late thirties to early forties.

According to the National Multiple Sclerosis Society, the condition affects approximately 400,000 Americans and 2.5 million people worldwide. About 200 new cases of MS are diagnosed each week. Multiple sclerosis is generally not considered a fatal disease.

Doctors still don't understand what causes multiple sclerosis. There is interesting and conflicting data that suggest that it could be caused by genetics, a person's environment, a virus, vascular issues, or even vitamin deficiencies.

Researchers believe that MS may be inherited and passed on from parents to children. Siblings of an affected person have a higher risk of developing MS. It's also found more often in twins.

The onset of multiple sclerosis may be severe or so mild that a person doesn't even notice any symptoms. Symptoms of multiple sclerosis vary from person to person and can change over time.

The most common early symptoms of MS include the following:

- Muscle weakness in one or more limbs (I had this.)
- Numbness and tingling in one or more limbs (I had this.)
- Loss of balance (I had this.)
- Blurred or double vision (I had optic neuritis)
- Eye pain (I had this.)
- Slurred speech
- Chronic fatigue (I had this for many months before I was diagnosed and throughout the years.)
- Lack of coordination (I had this.)

According to the National MS Society, as the disease progresses, symptoms may include the following:

* Fatigue is a *very* common characteristic of MS. It may consist of increased muscle weakness, mental fatigue, sleepiness, or drowsiness. The physical exhaustion that is felt is not related to the amount of activity; in fact, many patients with MS complain of extreme fatigue even after a good night's sleep. It's as if you wake up, and instead of being recharged and refreshed, you feel as if you didn't sleep at all. I used to hate that feeling. (This forced me to take two to three naps a day.)

* Dizziness causes many people with MS to complain of feeling "off balance" or lightheaded. Occasionally, they may experience vertigo—the feeling that their surroundings are spinning. (I had this when I was first diagnosed—that was one of the worst feelings I ever experienced.)

* Heat may worsen symptoms—high outdoor temperatures, hot showers, baths, or even in some cases, high levels of humidity. Heat sensitivity occurs in most people with MS. It will cause many people to feel "off" or dizzy, it may create numbness or tingling, and it may affect your arms or legs. (I used to have this a lot.)

* Cold can also worsen symptoms—cold temperatures, cold water, and even snow may affect some people. Symptoms may be the same as for heat sensitivity. The cold never affected me with worsening symptoms.

* Gait challenges are among the most common symptoms of MS due to muscle weakness or muscle spasms. Drop foot is also common. Having balance problems or numbness in your feet and legs can also make walking difficult. (I had this issue too; it's hard to walk when you can't feel your feet.)

* Vision problems are also very common. In fact, optic neuritis occurs very frequently. This can result in blurring or graying of

vision or even blindness in one eye. (This is actually how I came about being diagnosed with MS. I did not need new glasses, as my parents thought; it was optic neuritis.)

- Problems with thinking and cognition are a real challenge for people with MS. Brain fog can mean slowed thinking, decreased concentration, and severe memory issues. This can also decrease your ability to carry out your everyday tasks. (This is a real symptom of MS, and you're not just being slow or lazy. Some people around you may think you are faking or crazy, but it is normal, and you can have good days and bad days.)

- Muscle spasms are very common.

- Many of us living with MS experience abnormal or odd sensations such as pins and needles, numbness, itching, burning, stabbing, or tearing pains. (I used to have tearing pains in both my wrists, numbness and pins and needles in my feet and legs, also the feeling of electricity/tingling up my back.)

- People with MS can have swallowing difficulties. Speech problems can also occur.

Remember, many of these issues can happen on the inside, so others will not understand what you are going through for that reason.

CHAPTER 3

Top MS Myths

MS MYTHS HAVE THE POTENTIAL to completely derail someone by setting false expectations. In my experience, the following are the most common MS myths that are being shared throughout our communities today. If we are going to take charge of our health and our lives, it is important that we do not buy into these MS myths. We must protect our thoughts and create our beliefs based on truth, because the first step in recovering and living a healthy, productive life is believing in what is possible and not believing in ideas that will limit you.

MS myths are simply someone else's ideas, opinions, or projections. I have personally been able to defy these common MS myths, and I believe you can too.

MS MYTH 1: YOU DON'T LOOK SICK

If you look healthy on the outside—you walk normally, your skin looks normal, and your face appears normal—some may think that you're not sick and that you just complain all the time. Some may even think that you are faking symptoms for sympathy or that you are lazy and seeking support! This is not true.

MS is notorious for wreaking internal havoc on the body, starting from the top of your head to the tips of your toes. This is all unnoticeable on the outside, but it's very apparent to the MS sufferer. MS can be called one of the most silent or invisible disabilities because of this. With this common misconception, people are hurt over and over because of lack of understanding by others. The best thing we can do is to share information so we can change this type of thinking once and for all.

MS MYTH 2: YOU WILL DIE FROM MS

People don't have to die from MS itself. I know this is a point of contention because some will say they know people who have died from MS, but when you start to look at the cases, questions arise. Did they die from MS or from side effects from the MS drugs? Or did they die from a secondary infection or secondary condition? (I get it; MS can shut down the functioning of certain organs and systems in our bodies due to its progression, but with what I know now, it doesn't have to be like that for anyone!)

The good news is that people with MS can live just as long as anybody else. Sometimes, people who are very badly affected may get more infections or pick up other illnesses more easily than healthy people because of their compromised immune systems. But you *can* live just as long as anybody else. When I learned how to fix my body and heal my immune system, I understood this concept. You have that same control over your health!

MS MYTH 3: YOU SHOULDN'T HAVE CHILDREN

A woman with MS is less likely to have a relapse during pregnancy. (I myself had some of my healthiest times while I was pregnant.) However, the risk of relapse does increase in the months after the birth, due to the trauma of labor on your body. (I did have a relapse after having my first child, and I experienced loss of sensation and muscle control in my arms, specifically my hands, chronic fatigue, and also Bell's palsy.) Pregnancy has no long-term effect on MS, and you are no more likely to experience miscarriage, stillbirth, birth defects, or infant death than anyone else. When I had my second child, I suffered *no* relapses at all after his birth. I'm thrilled that I have been able to have two wonderful children, and it has been such a blessing to not only me, but my whole family. My twin sister, Kim, also has two beautiful children. If you're thinking about having children, please do your due diligence. There's lots of information out there about how you can have a safe, healthy, and happy pregnancy with MS. Be sure to discuss your family goals with your doctors.

At this point, I must share about my two pregnancies. My daughter, Sarah, was born in 1995; I was healthy and strong throughout the whole pregnancy. A few months after I had her, I had a bad flare-up. This was when I was following standard MS protocols. My son, Gregory, was born in 2005. I was healthy, strong, and active throughout the pregnancy, and after my son's birth, I had absolutely no issues or flare-ups. This was when I was following holistic and alternative therapies. Boy, what a difference!

MS Myth 4: You Cannot Work if You Have MS

MS is different for each person. Every person experiences different symptoms at different times, and the impact of the symptoms on your working life will very much depend on the type of work you do, your physical condition, and your own personal experience with MS. Some people might tell you to stop working right away after your diagnosis, but I believe you should continue as long as you can, if it's not too stressful. (You know, the whole idea that a body in motion stays in motion!) Many people with MS never experience severe enough symptoms to stop working. I worked for many years outside the home, and it was very rewarding. Being around great people just added to my life, personally and professionally. It is possible to have a good work life with MS. My employer knew of my diagnosis, and so did my coworkers, and I found that *most* employers were very compassionate and understanding. That being said, when my MS was at its worst, I did start working from home more than sixteen years ago. That gave me the security and freedom I needed. No matter what my MS was doing, being at home gave me the flexibility I desired, and it also gave me a connection with great people, which always kept my spirits up.

MS Myth 5: MS Isn't a Physically Painful Condition

MS patients do experience significant pain, although its severity fluctuates at any given time. Because symptoms change and vary so much from person to person, day to day, and month to month, it's impossible to diagnose or determine a person's levels of pain at any given time. This is hard for most people to understand, as it's happening internally to the person with MS. This was always tough, because people may think when you say you're hurting that you're faking it. Because to others, you look normal. Understand that you're not alone; MS can be painful, and this is something that anyone living with the disease can attest to. We can only hope to share information so that others can become aware of these types of issues with pain and hopefully be more aware and supportive.

MS Myth 6: You Can't Exercise with MS

Exercise is actually one of the most important activities to do, as it is helpful in managing so many of our MS symptoms. It's also important for our long-term health and well-being. Those who participate in any type of exercise program have better cardiovascular health, improved strength, better bladder and bowel function, less fatigue and depression, better sleep, and more positive attitudes. Many studies have confirmed the benefits of exercise (www.nationalmssociety.org). I myself have done many forms of exercise—weightlifting, Pilates, yoga, and aerobic activities—since I was a teenager.

Inactivity in people with or without MS can result in numerous challenges, including muscle weakness, cardiovascular disease, decreased bone density, shallow and inefficient breathing, bladder and bowel problems, fatigue, and depression. You have to think about it as a body in motion stays in motion. When you slow down or are inactive, it will greatly affect your health.

An exercise program needs to be appropriate to your own capabilities and any limitations you have. You know your body, and you should always pay attention to how you are feeling and what you are experiencing. Your activities may need to be adjusted as changes occur in your MS symptoms. Any person with MS who is initiating a new exercise program should also consult with his or her physician before starting. I know some people with MS also work out with trainers, who may not have a clue about MS. What I've found, in many cases, is that the trainer puts the person with MS on cardio activities like bike riding, walking, or even running on the treadmill. These are things that I will caution you about if you are having any issues with your legs or feet. In fact, when I was having the numbness, tingling, and pain issues with my legs, I did not go on the bike at all and greatly limited my time on the treadmill. If you fatigue your legs, you are doing a disservice to your body, and your symptoms may get worse. Once I was healing and strong, I could go on the bike and the treadmill with no problems. So really listen to your body and do something else, like lifting weights or swimming in a pool—things with little to no impact. Another note about trainers: if they are not familiar with MS and the overheating issues we have, they can push you beyond your limit, which is just not safe. So if you're looking to work out with a trainer, try to find one who is familiar with MS.

MS Myth 7: We Will Have a Cure in Five Years (or in Our Lifetime)

The most recent information that will have a huge impact on the course of MS is the fact that the National MS Society and the University of Iowa just committed over one million dollars to support clinical trials led by Dr. Terry Wahls (who overcame her own MS through diet and nutrition) to compare two popular MS diets, The Wahls protocol and The Swank Diet, to treat multiple sclerosis–related fatigue (www. nationalmssociety.org August 26, 2016). So that's definitely a point in the right direction.

In regard to the medical community and finding our cure, I will honestly say that I am hopeful, but I am very skeptical and concerned that most medical agencies are still predominantly focusing on drug therapy to achieve any kind of treatment for us. (In 1988, my pediatric neurologist said, "Don't worry, Kellie; there will be a cure for MS in five years.") Yes, that was back in 1988. I'm asking everyone to think about this realistically. Are we any closer to a cure now through traditional MS treatments?

We do have a plethora of drugs that only treat symptoms, and we have many more coming out, but what about something to repair our bodies and our immune systems? What about stopping the disease from ever happening in the first place? What about healing our whole body so MS is never an issue again?

There is new research and information every day that is changing the face of MS, and I believe it is the road to our cure. This information is coming from many different independents outside of traditional MS medicine—people who see that we need to treat our whole bodies, including the food we eat, the water we drink, our activity levels, the environments we live in, the things we think about, and the relationships we have. I'm hopeful and confident that we will find a cure outside of traditional medicine. I know I have found the pieces to the puzzle to heal my body!

MS myth #7 is exactly the reason we need to take personal responsibility for our own health and why we need to keep searching for information and supporting the pioneers who are leading the charge to cure our disease naturally.

CHAPTER 4

Just Say No

"Drugs are not always necessary, but belief in recovery always is."

—*Norman Cousins*

Disease-Modifying-Drug Debate

Yes, the old television commercials, school campaigns, and drug-free movements started such a memorable quote. You already know what that means: "Just say no to drugs," right?

Well, I'm really interested in talking to you about MS drugs and questions we should be asking ourselves and, of course, our doctors. Remember, I wrote this book to be thought-provoking, and I will be sharing plenty of ideas and theories, as well as my own questions and information in my quest to help you.

Since I have been dealing with MS for so long, I feel I have been around the proverbial block, if you will. Since I have been healthy, I have started to ask my own questions. After learning what I know now, I can't understand why the medical community has tried to continue to teach us that we must, must, must suppress our immune systems at all costs. Not only do doctors want us to suppress our immune systems, but in some cases, they ask us to take the most radical, harmful drugs in order to achieve that goal; this is just a question I'm asking.

Many MS patients have now taken more passive roles in their treatment of multiple sclerosis instead of looking to things that they can control, like diet, supplements, exercise, smoking choices, environments, relationships, and alternative therapies. What has evolved is an MS community that is predominantly focused on drug therapy and is made up of people who trust their medical professionals blindly. A lot of their health decisions are based on fear and lack of information.

Below is a list of Disease Modifying Drugs (DMDs) that are currently approved by the FDA. A name you may hear a lot in the drug arena is CRAB drugs, which stands for Copaxone, Rebif, Avonex, and Betaseron. These are considered the go-to drug therapies. There are always new ones coming on the horizon, or you may be using something that I didn't cover, but these are the most popular.

BETA INTERFERONS
Beta interferons are drugs such as Avonex, Betaseron, Extavia, and Rebif. If you are taking these, you will be warned about being around people who are sick. Interferons' side effects include: liver damage, so you'll need blood tests to monitor your liver enzymes; flu-like symptoms are the most common reaction, as well as injection-site reactions. (I remember my sister being very ill from this, in fact; her fever shot up to 105 degrees on a few occasions.) You may also have lower thyroid function and blood-cell abnormalities. You may also suffer from depression and anxiety. (nationalmssociety.org/diseasemodifyingmedications.)

COPAXONE
Copaxone can cause flushing and shortness of breath after injection. This drug may also take up to nine months to reach full effectiveness. It can also leave itchy, painful welts, and it may cause lipoatrophy (indention or depression in the skin and underlying tissue, which may

be permanent, due to injections.) You could have long-term flu-like symptoms. Copaxone also weakens your immune system. I've known several people who have almost died from simple infections because their bodies were so weakened by this DMD. (www.copaxone.com)

TYSABRI

Tysabri side effects include wheezing, chest pain, nose and throat infections, stomach pain, vaginitis, urinary-tract infections, lung infections, joint pain, and aches and pains in the limbs. Tysabri is supposed to be reserved for people who see no results from or can't tolerate other types of treatments, meaning this would be the last drug given in a series after other medications. However, I'm learning that more and more doctors are using this as a first step in treating MS, and that's just scary! This is because Tysabri increases the risk of progressive multifocal leukoencephalopathy (PML), which is a brain infection that is usually *fatal*. That's the worst-case scenario, but in my opinion, why take something that has the possibility of being fatal when we have so many other options and alternatives? (www.tysabri.com)

NOVANTRONE

Novantrone (Mitoxantrone) was only used to treat certain forms of cancer prior to its approval for use in MS. This drug can be harmful to the heart, and it's associated with development of blood cancers like leukemia, so it's usually only used to treat the most severe, advanced cases of multiple sclerosis. Why are we taking something that can give us cancer? (www.nationalmssociety.org/treating-MS/Novantrone)

GILENYA

Gilenya is a drug that can drastically slow your heartbeat, so you'll need to have your heart rate monitored for six hours after the first dose. Other side effects include headaches, flu-like symptoms, coughing, dizziness, high blood pressure, and visual blurring. There also have been cases of PML (progressive multifocal leukoencephalopathy) which is usually *fatal.* (www.gilenya.com)

Baclofen

Baclofen's side effects may include drowsiness, muscle weakness, dizziness or lightheadedness, confusion, constipation, unusual bladder symptoms, trouble sleeping, unusual unsteadiness or clumsiness, low blood pressure, and seizures. I know of an MS sufferer who was on this for muscle spasms. She had no previous issues with falling, but she had a severe reaction of muscle weakness and muscle failure in her legs; she would just fall at random times and without warning. She thought it was definitely a side effect of taking this. (www.nationalmssociety.org/treating-MS/Lioresal.com)

Tecfidera

Tecfidera may cause serious side effects. It decreases your white-blood-cell count and it can also cause progressive multifocal leukoencephalopathy, PML, the brain infection that usually leads to death or severe disability. Your doctor may check your white-blood-cell count before you take Tecfidera and from time to time during treatment. The most common side effects of Tecfidera include flushing and stomach problems. These can happen especially at the start of treatment and may decrease over time.

One interesting fact I need to share is that when I first started writing this book in 2012, I was investigating the newest MS drugs. One drug in particular, Tecfidera, had just been released and approved by the FDA. At that time, the drug's side effects were said to be minute and benign, if any. Well, fast-forward four years, and they now list the worst possible side effect, PML, the brain infection that can kill you. *Hmm*, I thought to myself, *how did this even get approved in the first place?* (www.tecfidera.com)

AUBAGIO

Aubagio has side effects that include severe liver problems, including death. Other side effects may include influenza, hair loss, nausea, diarrhea, and a reduced white-blood-cell count, which can definitely cause you to have more infections, and it can cause numbness or tingling in your hands and feet that is not caused by your MS. (Hmm, how can you tell it's different?) And why would you take something that may give you numbness and tingling if you didn't have it in the first place? Aubagio can also give you serious skin problems and high blood pressure.

All of the information I shared above is from the drug manufacturers' own websites and the National MS Society website. Although they say a certain drug may work in testing, to me that is just a small part of the big picture, and I am skeptical of any test results, because the drug companies make billions and billions of dollars off of each drug.

Yes, I covered a long list of side effects for each DMD. That was deliberate. I'm not trying to scare you; I want you to understand the risks associated with each one. I also wanted you to understand that deciding to use DMDs should not be taken lightly, and they could end up taking a lot from you. I also wonder whether after taking any DMD, if symptoms are from MS or just common drug side effects. Who could tell?

I have known many MS sufferers who are so debilitated and desperate, they are willing to do just about anything to be healed. I have talked with hundreds of MS sufferers who have said they really didn't want to know the DMD side effects, that it's just too scary; they will trust whatever their doctor tells them. I feel there are not enough people in the medical community sharing information about how to heal and treat your MS without the standard MS protocols. I feel we sometimes give away all our free will to the medical community, and in the long run, we hurt ourselves, as we have to pay for it financially and physically.

I also take the perspective that you don't know what you don't know. I didn't even know healing was possible, and that is why I'm writing about the possibility that you may get better and perhaps even conquer your MS. Because once you know, you can do something about it.

I'm glad we now have the new study being led by Dr. Terry Wahls focusing on nutrition and MS. It's a step in the right direction. Still, most doctors only talk about drug therapy and will tear down anything we may use to treat our MS that is in the realm of natural, holistic, or alternative.

Do your homework, talk with your doctor, and see what plan of attack is best for you. Or better yet, seek out a holistic or functional medical doctor; these professionals will have an entirely different spin on your disease, the ways to treat it, and how to heal your entire body!

My mantra is "A healthy immune system equals a healthy body."

I know the school of thought is to shut down the immune system so it stops attacking our bodies, but what if we work on having our immune system functioning properly? Doesn't that seem like a more viable long-term solution?

MS, when knocked down to its most simplistic state, is caused by inflammation or a breakdown of some sort in our bodies. Doesn't it make sense to engage in a lifestyle that would give our bodies' anti-inflammatory and healing benefits? I know some people believe MS is a vascular disease, some think it's an autoimmune issue, and some consider it a vitamin deficiency. Well, I respect your beliefs, whatever they are. I treated my MS as a vitamin deficiency and later as a need to heal my immune system, and that is how I came up with my plan of attack.

I was shocked that in all this time living with MS, none of my doctors ever mentioned alternatives to drug therapy. I was wondering whether it was because they just didn't know or whether they were manipulated in some way by Big Pharma. I mean, we know diet is important to our overall health, whether you have a health challenge like MS or not. That's common sense. Why aren't we given all the information, all the resources, all the alternatives, and all the possibilities so we can choose what the best course is for our own health and the best course of action for treating our disease?

Many people reading this might be on DMDs, and if you are, I hope and pray they are helping you. Again, I am writing this book to be thought-provoking and beneficial to you!

Here are some questions I have about any of the drugs used in traditional MS treatments:

- Will it cure my MS?
- Will it fight off the progression?
- Will it hurt my overall health long term?
- Will it suppress my immune system?
- Will I have to be on other drugs, too? (e.g., for pain, spasms, infections or depression)
- Can I ever get off the drugs?
- How long do the dmd's stay in our systems if we stop using?
- Can the drug(s) cause death?

The more profoundly a drug suppresses our immune functions, the more likely it will have very severe side effects!

I am also wondering whether there will ever be a time when drug therapy will not be standard for every person. When you start investigating all the MS drugs, their costs, and the profits Big Pharma and our doctors make from them, you can't help but take a step back and wonder whether the medical community really wants to find a cure. We're talking about billions and billions of dollars in profits from MS drugs. It's definitely something to think about.

In conclusion, whether you continue using MS drugs or decide to just say no, you and your doctor should map out a plan for what is best for you by looking at a variety of factors.

* Effectiveness
* Safety
* Cost
* Side effects
* Long-term health concerns stemming from use

I do believe in the use of steroids to get over a flare-up. I think it's a necessary part of this healing process, but after the steroid treatments, it's essential to do everything possible to lessen inflammation in the body and really focus on healing.

I hope you realize that you have options, and you have an obligation to yourself to know any and all information that can affect your disease. I know that once I started focusing on my options, things started to come together, and I believe it saved my life.

I've talked previously about my twin sister, Kim. Well, I watched her take all the CRAB drugs and a few others too—and what I witnessed was constant illness, more exacerbations, and a full progression of her disease. (All this happened while I was virtually symptom-free by following alternatives to heal.)

CHAPTER 5

Environmental Toxins

"It is horrifying that we have to fight our own
government to save the environment."

—ANSEL ADAMS

ENVIRONMENTAL TOXINS CAN HAVE AN immediate effect on MS sufferers. They can bring on exacerbations, and compromise both our immune and nervous system. With MS, we have to look at the body as a whole. There is not one specific thing that will heal us. We need to look at actions and steps we can take cumulatively to heal our bodies and inevitably heal our immune systems.

SMOKING

This is a self-inflicted toxin, and in most cases, it can be avoided either by quitting smoking or by staying away from secondhand smoke. Smoking is very debilitating. In fact, if someone with MS has even a few puffs of a cigarette, he or she can have an exacerbation. It's that harmful! The risk of developing MS doubles for people who smoke. The toxic substances in a cigarette may also put an MS sufferer at risk for progressing the whole disease process. In MRIs, smokers showed more brain lesions than non-smokers (www.mssociety.org/smoking).

It's also interesting to look at the flip side—that MS symptoms could be the exact reason some reach for a cigarette. Think about it—some experience depression, anxiety, stress, and fatigue. I know that many people who smoke and have a debilitating condition like MS may actually lack support and understanding from others. People will say, "You're doing it to yourself by smoking." It's totally self-inflicted, but no matter what, we should stop blaming people for what they choose to do. MS sufferers still need friendship, understanding, and support. Do you know anyone who smokes and has MS? Are you the one who has MS and still smokes? My sister smokes; she's stopped and started many times. I've thrown away her cigarettes out of frustration—you see, I just want her to be healthy. I know that's a rough tactic, but I was taking the stance of tough love. My heartfelt tip is that you should stop smoking immediately, and try to avoid secondhand smoke too.

Here are some interesting facts about smokers:

- Smokers are diagnosed with MS younger than non-smokers.
- Smokers are more likely to get MS than non-smokers.
- Smokers tend to have more lesions than non-smokers.

MERCURY

Mercury is one of the worst toxic metals. Mercury is in some dental fillings, and the fillings are not only toxic as they sit in your mouth, but each time you eat, they release mercury into your body. Mercury crosses the blood-brain barrier and negatively affects our central nervous system (CNS). Mercury toxicity can cause serious health problems. Not only can it cause many neurological issues like MS, it can also cause cancer. There is a lot of controversy surrounding whether or not to get your fillings removed. It's not a simple procedure, since extracting the fillings will put mercury into the air, and it can be a danger to the doctor and the patient. So it's important to do your research, talk to a specialist, and then analyze whether this is the proper step for you to take. I know of several people who have had this done successfully.

Mercury is also widely used as thimerosal, a toxic mercury-based preservative in vaccines, including flu vaccines, and it is not safe. High concentrations of mercury can also be found in some fish, including swordfish, king mackerel, shark, marlin, and tuna.

If you're concerned about mercury levels in your body, you may want to be tested to see whether your mercury levels are high enough to cause any health concern. It is normal to find trace amounts of mercury in the body, and a test may show that you don't have anything to worry about. To get rid of mercury in your body, many people use chelation therapy as well as different vitamin therapies. The great news is that you have options. While mercury may not be the sole cause of MS, addressing mercury toxicity efficiently may resolve a great number of symptoms. Remember, we have to look at many different factors to assess how to heal our entire bodies. I am personally on a vitamin chelation therapy because when I had my mercury levels tested, they were elevated.

Sodium Lauryl Sulfate (SLS)

Sodium lauryl sulfate (SLS) is a foaming agent used in most toothpaste, shampoo, shaving cream, bubble bath, mouthwash, moisturizer, detergent, and cleaners. It can cause skin irritation and rashes, eye irritation, and even hair loss. In toothpaste, SLS has been linked to canker sores. Swallowing SLS can cause nausea and diarrhea. This is easy enough to fix simply by starting to read labels and getting products that are SLS-free. Remember, we are trying to heal our bodies. Any toxins we can avoid will only help our immune systems.

Air Pollution

"Fall is my favorite season in Los Angeles, watching
the birds change color and fall from the trees."

—David Letterman

In areas with poor air quality, MS exacerbation rates are much higher. Nowadays, children and adults are spending up to 90 percent of their time indoors, and our modern homes are sealed airtight. Indoor air, in particular, can be five to ten times more polluted than outdoor air. Looking at indoor air quality and how it may be a factor in an MS flare-up is very interesting. Pollutants or particulates in the air can cause immune challenges, and they can also affect our nervous systems.

When you look around your home, you can see many things that may be contributing factors, such as off-gassing from carpets (formaldehyde). Paints can bother the eyes and lungs and even affect the nervous system. (Paints can emit VOCs, or volatile organic compounds, so it's important to buy paints that are low in VOCs.) Nail polishes, nail-polish removers, glues, whiteboard markers, furniture pieces made from particle or pressed boards that contain formaldehyde; indoor cleaning products; air fresheners; laundry detergents; fabric softeners; fabric-softener sheets; even candles can cause indoor air pollution. Viruses and bacteria can also be polluting your air, which makes MS sufferers even more susceptible to illnesses, infections, and exacerbations.

I want to remind you that there is not a one-step, quick-fix solution to heal our bodies and our immune systems, but a culmination of steps will help to ensure our overall health.

Air quality is really a twofold challenge, as we have to focus on the outdoor air and also our indoor air quality. I recommend checking out the American Lung Association's website for the most updated air-quality reports for your city.

We need to ensure that the air we breathe is not filled with particulates, pollutants, and contaminants. This is why I highly recommend a whole-home air-purification system. My family also uses air purifiers when we travel.

WATER POLLUTION

"Water is life's mother and medium. There is no life without water!"

—ALBERT SZENT-GYORGYI

I once heard a speaker talk about water and that one day, it will rule the world, meaning that whoever controls or can provide fresh, clean water will control everything. Is that a fair statement? I think it is. It's essential for everyone. We need to have clean, healthy water that is free of toxins, chemicals, and bacteria to ensure our bodily systems can function properly. The challenge is that our water systems in the United States are old, outdated, and unprepared for the future.

Tap water is a huge problem, according to the Environmental Working Group (EWG). Testing that has been done in the last decade has shown more than three hundred different pollutants in the tap water Americans drink. More than half of the chemicals detected in drinking water are not subject to health or safety regulations. These findings pose huge challenges for utilities that are detecting dozens of unregulated substances in treated drinking water, including pharmaceutical drugs and industrial chemicals that pass unfiltered through conventional treatment methods. Chromium, lead, and fluoride can be found in high levels around the nation and are known carcinogens.

Do you remember the movie *Erin Brockovich* with Julia Roberts? (She won an Oscar for that performance.) The movie was based on a true story. Erin Brockovich finds a cover-up in Hinkley, California, and learns that the drinking water was polluted by hexavalent chromium. The residents of Hinkley had tons of medical problems, tumors, cancers, etc. The story revolved around her proving that the mega company PG&E knew about the groundwater poisoning from the hexavalent chromium, and a legal battle ensued. This is not an isolated incident. The issues with chromium are rampant across the United States. I know the water in Chicago is filled with different chemicals, including lead, chlorine, fluoride, pharmaceuticals, PCE (dry-cleaning chemicals and industrial cleaners), and pesticides.

FLUORIDE
Fluoride is added to many water supplies around the country to supposedly help us, but it's dangerous. It's a known carcinogen and neurotoxin. It does not help your teeth, and it will accumulate in your body. It can lead to issues in your brain and nervous system. It can cause arthritis, reduced thyroid function, autoimmune challenges, and even cancer. I recommend checking out the Fluoride Action Network online for the latest news and information about the specific challenges associated with any intake of fluoride. It's not safe. We need to protect ourselves from any chemicals, specifically ones that cross the blood-brain barrier.

LEAD
Another big concern about our water supply is lead. We've heard about the lead-tainted water in Flint, Michigan, and now throughout Chicago's school systems. This water is not safe and cannot be used in any form. These are not isolated incidents. *USA Today* did its own investigation called "Lead in Your Water" (www.usatoday.com) and

found over two thousand water systems around the United States that showed high levels of lead contamination. The challenges with lead in our water supplies come from outdated pipes that would cost billions of dollars to update. Lead can damage our nervous systems, reproductive systems, and kidneys, cause learning disabilities, and even cause cancer.

A great resource for the most updated health information is the Environmental Working Group's website (EWG.org). You can go to that website and check out the water quality in your area.

I highly recommend getting a water purifier—not only to ensure your drinking water is safe, but also to ensure you are drinking enough clean, healthy water every day. Water consumption is significant for MS sufferers because many MS symptoms get worse from lack of water. In fact, dehydration can mimic many MS symptoms, including fatigue, dizziness, headaches, aches, and pains.

BOTTLED WATER

Bottled water is also another big issue. In the last decade, consumers have been drinking millions of gallons of bottled water. Many people have switched over to bottled water, believing that it is actually safer than tap water. Many plastic bottles and food-storage containers contain BPA (bisphenol A), which is an industrial chemical that has been used to make certain plastics and resins since the 1960s.

BPA is a known neurotoxin and carcinogen. When BPA is ingested, it has been found to impair neurological functions and even cause cancer. The EWG conducted a study that found BPA had dissolved into half of the randomly selected canned foods, water bottles, and beverages they tested. (www.ewg.org/bpa).

There also have been conflicting reports as to the true source of natural spring water. The EWG conducted comprehensive testing on some popular brands of U.S. bottled water and found contaminants, including the following:

- Cancer-causing byproducts of chlorination
- Fertilizer residues, such as nitrate and ammonia
- Industrial solvents
- Caffeine
- Pharmaceuticals, such as Tylenol, birth-control pills, and heart medicines
- Heavy metals and minerals, including arsenic and radioactive chemicals
- Other industrial chemicals

The bottled water tested contained thirty-eight chemical pollutants altogether, with an average of eight contaminants in each brand. More than one-third of the chemicals found are not regulated. (www.ewg.org/research/bottled-water-quality)

Plastic bottles can also be carcinogenic. Plastics have a high incidence of bacterial contamination. This means these bottles should never be refilled, especially if left in warm temperatures. Also, the water from these bottles should not be used after sitting without refrigeration.

Years ago famous musician Sheryl Crow went on *Larry King Live* and stated that she is compelled to educate people about not drinking out of plastic water bottles that have been sitting in the car. If it gets hot, it's emitting byproducts that can cause cancer, she warned (CNN *Larry King Live*, aired August 23, 2006). Bottled water being unhealthy after sitting for days in heat seems like a logical conclusion to me too, but many bottled-water companies and even some doctors are stating that the theory is not true. You can do your own research and be the judge of what you think is best for you and your family.

The bottom line is that we need to ensure we are drinking enough water to combat dehydration, and we need to make sure it's healthy, pure water! There are plenty of great water-purification systems on the market to help. I have been using an awesome water technology and have been doing so for almost sixteen years. It allows me to drink and cook with alkaline, pH-balanced water, which helps me stay hydrated and helps flush toxins out of my body. I also use a special filtered water pitcher that takes out fluoride, heavy metals, and other known chemicals. I also use filters in my shower.

The EWG website has a comprehensive list of bottled waters; check it out, and see where yours ranks.

Parabens

Parabens are preservatives found in many cosmetics, skin- and body-care products, antiperspirants, deodorants, suntan lotions, and even some drugs. You may see one or more of the following on a product's label—methylparaben, propylparaben, isopropylparaben, isobutylparaben, and sodium butylparaben. To make looking at labels easier, notice any ingredient that ends with "paraben"—that's the issue. The challenge with parabens is that they have been found to mimic estrogen. Some people think this can be a possible trigger for cancer, especially breast cancer. There is no safety testing on these ingredients.

We must become avid label readers to ensure the products we are using do not have carcinogens in them, and we need to make sure we limit our exposure as much as possible to these agents, since they may compromise our immune systems.

Remember, healing is about treating the body as whole.

We can help to ensure our good health by reading labels and buying organic or all-natural products. Because of the whole, healthy, green movement today, it's easier to buy these products locally. You can purchase items from Whole Foods, Trader Joe's, many specialty health stores, and you can even find everything online; just Google what you are specifically looking for.

I shop at many different stores; it's nice to have relationships with business owners who can tell you about new products and new information that may be of benefit to you and your particular condition.

MOLD

Mold is very much a hidden issue. Many people don't realize they have a mold problem, let alone mold toxicity, but it can be deadly. Mold can be worse than pesticides and heavy metals in damaging the body. Mold toxicity can be the cause of many psychological and neurological disorders such as anxiety, bipolar disorder, chronic fatigue, depression, fibromyalgia, insomnia, cancer, even multiple sclerosis.

Mold toxicity is commonly misdiagnosed. It should be of great concern to all of us, because mold toxins can destroy the myelin sheath in the brain.

There are many holistic doctors who do mold testing and treatment. The doctor may have you do a skin, blood, or urine test. I highly recommend looking into being tested for mold toxicity, as its symptoms closely mimic many MS symptoms. And remember, long-term mold toxicity can actually cause MS. That's really scary! If we can eliminate that as a cause, we can then focus on other areas for healing. I had mold-toxicity testing and was glad to find out that it's not an issue for me.

One point I want to reiterate is that having MS is complex. One specific thing didn't give us MS, and there won't be one factor or single step to our cure. We must be diligent in looking at many avenues for not only understanding our disease, but ways to beat it.

CHAPTER 6

Stress Test

"The life of inner peace, being harmonious and
without stress is the easiest type of existence."

—*Norman Vincent Peale*

THERE ARE MANY PHYSICAL, EMOTIONAL, and even financial challenges to having multiple sclerosis that can definitely contribute to both chronic and acute stress. *Merriam-Webster's Dictionary* defines stress as a negative concept that can have an impact on one's mental and physical well-being. One thing MS sufferers know all too well is that stress is toxic to us and our good health. Nowadays, it seems MS sufferers are overloaded with stressful situations and stressful lifestyles not only due to our disease, but also because of our overextended schedules, as we try to do everything and be everything to everyone. With MS, we have to be particularly mindful of stress, as it can be a contributing factor to our exacerbations. Yes, of course, daily living with MS can be very stressful due to the mere fact that we never know from day to day what will transpire. We could be hit with an exacerbation at any time—fatigue, brain fog, pain and physical challenges all come as part of dealing with this disease.

When you think about stress, each person has his or her own unique stressors. Some people will react to stressors by addressing them head-on, trying to solve the problems, while others will run away and just not deal with them at all. Stress can put us on high alert, and our bodies' natural response is to go into the fight-or-flight mode.

Have you ever been in a stressful situation? Did you notice anything happening within your body during that time? I have, and in stressful situations, I notice that my stomach starts churning, my heart starts beating at what seems like a thousand beats per minute, and I get a sudden burst of energy. The flip side of that fight-or-flight mode (and I've experienced that, too) is extreme sudden-onset fatigue—there's a definite crash-and-burn feeling of being wiped out. That is not healthy!

One thing I have discovered over the years is that if I did have a particularly stressful situation or life event, maybe even one that was a long-term, ongoing issue, I didn't have any flare-ups or experience health challenges until a few months later, when things had calmed down. Maybe you have experienced that too. That has happened to me on more than one occasion over the years. I was OK during the stressful time, but boom! Weeks or months down the line, I had a massive flare-up. (This was before switching over to alternatives and holistic treatments for my disease.)

The body is an incredible machine, and all its reactions are to protect us quickly and effectively for a short time. Problems come about when stress is ongoing. Our bodies are not meant to function in that capacity (fight or flight) for any significant length of time.

The changes our bodies undergo when we are stressed are well documented. You can have headaches, increased pain, dizziness, depression, IBS, elevated heart rate and blood pressure, sleeplessness, panic attacks, numbness, and immense fatigue.

Of course, the worst part of stress with MS is that it wreaks havoc on our immune systems, and in some cases, new lesions can develop. I cannot express more strongly how bad stress is for our bodies!

How Can We Tell If We Are Stressed?

* Do you suffer from headaches?
* Do you have upper G.I. issues?
* Do you suffer from chronic fatigue?
* Do you have trouble concentrating?
* Do you constantly worry?

* Are you overly negative?
* Do you over or under eat?
* Do you suffer from depression?
* Do you have a short temper?
* Are you moody?

If you answered yes to any of the items above, it's important to understand there are plenty of ways to address stress productively so you don't suffer negative health consequences.

Ways to beat stress and help your MS:

* Talk to a trusted friend/loved one
* Practice deep breathing
* Pray/meditate
* Acupuncture
* Watch a funny movie
* Read an uplifting book
* Write – affirmations, goals
* Play with a pet

* Join a support group
* Dance
* Listen to music
* Exercise – Pilates, yoga, weightlifting
* Get a massage
* Hypnosis
* Get into nature
* Smile

There are physiological responses that happen in our bodies from meditation, yoga, tai chi, breathing exercises, massage, and daily prayer - this can counteract damage from any chronic stress.

It's important not to negate your feelings of stress, anxiety, or depression; instead, talk to someone, such as a trusted friend or loved one who is not judgmental, who is willing to be a sounding board for you, and who can be supportive of what you are going through. As many of us know all too well, sometimes the people closest to us can hurt us the most by not being there for us. It's not that they don't care; it's that they simply do not understand what we are going through. Remember, MS is an invisible disease, as we may not be outwardly showing our current health challenges.

Find people who are also living with MS and can understand your plight. I'm on many different MS support-group sites on social media that are full of cutting-edge information; they are positive, uplifting, and focus on having the right perspective. It's important to talk with people who understand what we are going through. I highly recommend investigating the resources you have around your own area. You need to understand that you are not alone in this battle. We are in this together, and one by one, we can help support each other.

CAN OUR DIETS AFFECT OUR STRESS LEVELS?

Yes, our diets can affect our stress levels. Look for an anti-inflammatory diet; I will share specific information about the best diets for MS later in the book, below are some stress-fighting foods you can start on right away.

Stress fighting foods:

* Salmon (wild caught)
* Spinach
* Nuts
* Blueberries
* Green Tea
* Flax seed/Flax oil
* Avocado
* Sunflower seeds
* Asparagus
* Oatmeal
* Oranges
* Dark chocolate

Stress is something we can control, and once you start listening to your body, you will notice the changes that arise when you are in a particularly stressful situation. Try this: the next time you are in a stressful situation, stop, and notice what's happening to you. What are you feeling? What are you thinking? What is your body doing? At that point, you can step back momentarily, take a breath, and choose which one of the tools from above that you will use to de-stress.

Yes, change is sometimes difficult, but what is the alternative? We know stress can hurt us physically—if not right away, then definitely over time.

I remember that when my MS was really in overdrive, any stressful situation seemed to exhaust me. I would feel out of sorts and just washed out. I would feel as though I had been run over by a truck or had just run a marathon. I've also heard this type of feeling from my MS friends. This is a real reaction happening from stress. Learn to identify it so you can respond adequately to each situation.

Years ago, I wish I had some tips and techniques to help me calm down. The tips I shared above do continue to help me every day and have now become things I do without thinking. In a particularly rough situation, my subconscious will take over before I can have any of those negative side effects! In each stressful situation, I think about what is happening, what I want my end result to be, and finally, the best way to handle the challenge in the least stressful way. And since I've been symptom-free, stressful situations do not affect me like they used to. That gives me hope for others to be able to accomplish the same thing. I pray you can have the same type of results and benefits.

CHAPTER 7

You Are What You Eat

"Let food be thy medicine and medicine be thy food."

—HIPPOCRATES

WHAT KIND OF DIET SHOULD I FOLLOW?

I WAS ALWAYS A JUNK-FOOD junkie. I grew up right across the street from a candy store. Yes, all the allowance money for the kids in my neighborhood went to that store. I have many fond memories of long summer days walking with my friends, especially my best friend, Debbie, with our bags of candy in hand. I really never understood the correlation between eating healthy foods and being healthy. I didn't even understand how important supplements were to my diet. I was first introduced to a different kind of thinking in 2001, the thinking that actually changed my life: being healthy can be accomplished, and it is our responsibility to live the lives we were meant to live.

There's too much research showing that diet plays a major role in the initiation and even the progression of MS for us not to look at our diets and how they affect our health. Our highly processed, sugar-packed diets are, of course, unhealthy, and they lead to disease; we cannot sit back and just wonder about the correlation between eating right and the effects that it has on our MS.

In the pages below, I've included diets that are popular with people dealing with MS. Although I don't follow any particular diet, I have added and subtracted more foods than I can count.

The Overcoming MS Diet (OMS)

The OMS Recovery Program is based on the pillars of diet, exercise, stress management, sunlight, vitamin-D and omega-3 supplementation, and, when needed, medication. Here is a summary of the Overcoming Multiple Sclerosis Recovery Program:

Diet and supplements:

* A plant-based whole-food diet plus seafood, with no saturated fat, as far as is practical
* Omega-3 fatty-acid supplements (20–40 ml of flaxseed oil daily; fish oil can be substituted, if desired)
* Optional B-group vitamins or B-12 supplements, if needed

Vitamin D

* Get fifteen to twenty minutes of sunlight daily, three to five times a week
* Take a vitamin D-3 supplement of at least 5,000 IU daily, adjusted to blood level
* Aim to keep your blood level of vitamin D high, that is between 150–225 nmol/L (may require up to 10,000 IU daily)

MEDITATION

⟡   Thirty minutes daily

EXERCISE

⟡   Twenty to thirty minutes around five times a week, preferably outdoors

This is another fabulous recovery program that has helped many MS sufferers start to live healthy and productive lives.

("Improving Life with Multiple Sclerosis | Overcoming MS." *Overcoming MS Homepage Comments*. N.p., n.d. Web. 08 Nov. 2016.)

THE SWANK DIET

Dr. Roy Swank discovered that a diet very low in saturated fats and polyunsaturated oils helps MS patients live healthy and productive lives. The diet was formulated after fifty years of research following hundreds of patients. It's simple to follow and in many cases alleviates many chronic symptoms. This diet is supported by the MS Society and its doctors.

Here is a quick reference guide to the Swank Diet:

⟡   Processed foods containing saturated fats or hydrogenated oils are not permitted.
⟡   Saturated fat should not exceed 15 g per day. Unsaturated fat (oils) should be kept to between 20-50 g per day.
⟡   Fruits and vegetables are permissible in any amount.

- Red meat is not permitted for the first year, including pork. After the first year, 3 oz. of red meat is allowed once per week.
- White-meat, skinless poultry and white fish are permissible, but avoid dark-meat poultry and limit fatty fish to 50 g (1.75 oz.) per day.
- Dairy products must contain 1 percent or less butterfat unless otherwise noted. Use egg whites only (no yolks).
- Cod liver oil (1 tsp. or equivalent capsules) and a multivitamin and mineral supplement are recommended daily.
- Whole-grain breads, rice, and pastas are encouraged.
- Daily snacks of nuts and seeds are good sources of natural oils and help maintain good energy levels.

You can find the Swank Diet by visiting SwankMSDiet.org. I have many friends who are on this diet, and it has taken them from severe disabilities and living in a wheelchair to full mobility and much healthier, symptom-free lives.

("Swank MS Foundation: For Your Health, For Your Future." *Swank MS Foundation*. N.p., n.d. Web. 08 Nov. 2016.)

The Wahls Protocol

Dr. Terry Wahls overcame her secondary progressive MS (SPMS) by changing her diet. Her paleo diet took her from a wheelchair and being homebound to healthy. Dr. Wahls researched what nutrients we might need for maximum support of both our mitochondria and our brain cells. She is at the forefront of research based on diet and nutrition, not medication. I don't follow this diet, due to its focus on organ meats, higher-fat foods, and a few of the other items on the menu, but I agree with the information about adding fruits and greens, sulfur-rich foods, and the nutrients you need to have healthy cells. It is basic science about what our bodies need to heal.

(Wahls, Terry L., and Eve Adamson. *The Wahls Protocol: A Radical New Way to Treat all Chronic Autoimmune Conditions Using Paleo Principles.* New York: Avery, 2015. Print.)

Raw Diet

Following a raw diet means what you eat will be plant-based foods never heated above 115 degrees. Although I don't follow a raw diet (I like many of my foods cooked), I do love green juicing. I know many people who have overcome great health crises by going raw. Raw food is packed with enzymes and nutrients to make your body alkaline. If your body is in an alkaline state, it cannot harbor disease.

Raw food should be organic, meaning it should contain no pesticides and no GMOs (genetically modified organisms, which I'll explain in more detail later in the chapter)—and it should not be microwaved, processed, or cooked. When you overcook foods, especially vegetables, you take out the vitamins—the good stuff.

Some people follow a 100 percent raw diet. The initial detoxifying process can be very tough; however, you will get over that. Some people follow it only at 85 percent or even 50/50, but whatever way you choose to add raw foods to your diet, you can be very healthy, energized, and strong.

On the raw diet, you'll eat plenty of fresh vegetables, fresh fruits, eggs, seeds, nuts, raw nut butters, sprouted grains, lentils, fresh vegetable juices, and herbal teas. You may even consume sea veggies, fermented foods, or raw dairy products.

I have several friends on a raw diet, and they said if you follow this diet you should pay attention to your vitamin D and vitamin B-12 levels. They take supplements.

Vegetarian Diet

Generally speaking, vegetarians don't eat meat. However, there are a few different types of vegetarian diets. Vegans eat only plant foods. They stay away from any foods that come from animals. Lacto-vegetarians consume dairy products, but avoid eggs. Lacto-ovo-vegetarians consume dairy products and eggs.

One issue MS sufferers have to be aware of is any specific diet that advocates certain gluten-containing foods and certain grains that could raise insulin levels and lead to increased inflammation and the risk of more autoimmune challenges.

The Gluten Free Diet

There is a lot of information out there about going gluten free and healing your MS. For some, gluten free is the latest fad. Some people stop eating gluten due to illness; others are looking at what to cut out of their diets because of rising food allergies or sensitivities and even autoimmune diseases. Gluten is a protein that is found in wheat, barley, rye, and sometimes oats. When I think of gluten, I think of the word "glue." Gluten is just an unhealthy binder, and why would we want glue in our bodies?

Wheat (nearly all types of grain) rapidly turns into sugar in the body, causing spikes in our insulin levels that put our bodies into an inflammatory state. Inflammation in the body contributes to disease. Our Western diet is packed full of wheat, highly processed, genetically modified wheat foods, and unhealthy carbs. Wheat is capable of causing health problems like celiac disease, gluten intolerance, headaches, irritable-bowel syndrome, rheumatoid arthritis, asthma, cancers, and many autoimmune issues, including MS.

My best friends are gluten free due to celiac disease and gluten sensitivities, and they have the most flavorful and wide-ranging meals.

Going gluten free does not mean taste free; you can still use your spices and have foods that are healthy and full of flavor. Many restaurants now have gluten free menu options available.

One point to consider about going gluten free is that it does not automatically mean healthy; if you replace a regular cupcake with a gluten free cupcake, it's basically the same problem for an MS sufferer and, for that matter, anyone on this diet. Make sure the foods you are consuming aren't overly processed and full of unhealthy additives.

One other point, lots of gluten free diets use white rice as a staple, but this is also a highly processed grain that is converted into sugar as soon as you eat it, and it will cause inflammation. That is something MS sufferers should avoid.

The Dairy-Free Diet

There is mounting evidence that consumption of cow's milk is a contributing factor in the development of MS and other autoimmune diseases. Respected nutritionist and health researcher Dr. T. Colin Campbell reveals the truth about cow's milk in his best-selling book, *The China Study*. In this study, he shows direct links between MS and a number of other Western diseases from animal fat and protein, particularly from cow's milk ingestion. "People who ate the most animal-based foods got the most chronic disease. People who ate the most plant-based foods were the healthiest and tended to avoid chronic disease."

Most dairy products contain growth hormones. In fact, Monsanto's rBGH (recombinant bovine growth hormone) is a synthetic form of growth hormone injected into cows to increase their growth and milk production. (See more about Monsanto below.) Manufactured by Monsanto, rBGH has been banned in almost thirty countries, but it is still in most US cows. If you must drink milk, buy organic and limit dairy consumption. There is plenty of compelling information saying that for MS sufferers, milk may not do the body good! Campbell reports the correlation between consuming cow's milk and the incidence of MS.

(Campbell, T. Colin, and Thomas M. Campbell. *The China Study: The Most Comprehensive Study of Nutrition Ever Conducted and the Startling Implications for Diet, Weight Loss and Long-term Health.* Dallas, TX: BenBella, 2005. Print.)

> "The doctor of the future will no longer treat the human frame with
> drugs, but rather will cure and prevent disease with nutrition."
>
> —THOMAS EDISON

AN ANTI-INFLAMMATORY DIET

The first step to fight inflammation in the body can be to eat foods that are full of antioxidants, which are compounds that fight off free radicals that can damage our cells. Long-term damage to our cells can definitely lead to diseases like MS, even cancer.

Omega-3 fats are a potent anti-inflammatory nutrient. Yes, they help fight inflammation, but they're great for your heart's health, even brain and cognitive function; they can also help prevent autoimmune issues, cancers, and rheumatoid arthritis. Great sources of omega-3 fats are fatty fish like wild salmon and sardines, grass-fed meats, walnuts, wild rice, and flaxseed.

Foods that can reduce inflammation include red or white onions, tomatoes (if there is no sensitivity), broccoli, sweet potatoes, spinach, cucumbers, cauliflower, red grapes, berries, papayas, and oranges; these are all packed with anti-inflammatory properties.

Ginger, basil, cayenne, chives, cinnamon, garlic, rosemary, and turmeric, either dried or fresh, are among the healthiest spices and herbs.

Below are items you should use in moderation or try to avoid:

* Trans fats. Although many manufacturers are reducing or removing this type of fat, check out every label. You should never eat trans fats.
* White starches include flour, sugar, and white rice; these can cause quick spikes in blood-sugar levels, which put your body into an inflammatory state.
* Animal fats include red meat, poultry skin, and whole-milk dairy products. I limit my red-meat intake and limit my dairy consumption, always thinking about what causes inflammation.
* Avoid excess alcohol use. Limit your consumption to one or two alcoholic beverages a day or in one sitting; too much alcohol can trigger more unwanted inflammation and also affects your gut health.

The Organic Diet

The term "organic" refers to foods grown without synthetic pesticides, insecticides, herbicides, hormones, and other substances. It will not have added artificial flavors or colors. Organic meat, poultry, eggs, and dairy products come from animals that are not given antibiotics or growth hormones. Organic food is produced without using pesticides, bioengineering methods, or radiation.

We must pause here when talking about an organic diet, and I believe this has to do with our overall health. No matter what diet you are following—one of those I've listed above or perhaps something else— you must understand that GMOs, genetically modified organisms, altering genes through genetic engineering, is one of the worst processes ever used to destroy our healthy food supplies. Its long-term ramifications, not only to our health, but also to our planet, are being studied by the top doctors and scientists from around the world. Anything that can be labeled as a GMO is not healthy, and it's not safe!

What Are GMOs?
GMOs are plants or animals created through genetic engineering (GE). This is *experimental*, and I say "experimental" because we still don't know all the long-term effects genetic engineering will have on our health. Virtually all commercial GMOs are engineered to withstand the direct application of herbicides or to produce insecticides.

Recently, my son asked why the bugs are going after the organic corn in our garden, yet they are not touching any of the corn in the nearby fields. (We have several farms around us.) It's because the seeds now have an insecticide built in so bugs won't damage the crops.

Despite the promises from Monsanto, none of the GMO crops on the market offer increased crop yields or drought tolerance, enhanced nutrition, or any other consumer benefit. None at all!

Are GMOs Safe?
Many countries do not consider GMOs to be safe. As of this printing, almost seventy countries, including Australia, Japan, and even Russia have banned GMOs or have put significant restrictions on their production and sale.

In the United States, the government has approved GMOs based on studies conducted by Monsanto (yes, the same company that created these fake foods, if you will, and has then gained billions from their sale). Google "Monsanto" so you can understand the ramifications of GMO foods. The information is mounting and is available to all of us. We have to take matters into our own hands by buying organics and non-GMO foods. It's the only true way to take control of your diet and your health.

ARE GMOS LABELED?

Even though polls consistently show that Americans want to know whether the food they're purchasing contains GMOs, the biotech lobby has succeeded in keeping this information from us. You've probably heard about the DARK act, also known as the Deny Americans the Right to Know Act. This act is all about hiding what is in our foods. I found out much of this information from the Non-GMO Project; this organization was created to give consumers the informed choices we deserve. I'm an avid follower of the Non-GMO Project for the most updated and beneficial information (www.nongmo.org). I highly recommend getting involved in demanding the right to know what's in our foods.

Unfortunately, in August 2016, Congress approved and President Obama expanded Monsanto's control by signing the DARK Act. It will undo Vermont's GMO labeling law that was to be the standard for other states to follow in labeling all our foods. This is disturbing information and shows that the government is not concerned about protecting its citizens. They are controlled by big industries. This means you must become an avid label reader and investigator to try to understand food ingredients and what they mean to your health. I cannot imagine what our food supply will look like for future generations.

Avoiding pesticides and GMO foods will definitely help your MS. Chemicals and pesticides can hurt our nervous systems and cause widespread inflammation in our bodies, which will not only affect our MS, but can also cause cancer. Another key thing to point out is that just because something states it's non-GMO does not mean it's made without pesticides, heavy metals, hormones, sewage sludge, or other drug residues. So going organic is always the best way to avoid that.

Of all the top GMO foods, perhaps two of the most devastating ingredients to be added to our foods today are aspartame and MSG (monosodium glutamate).

Aspartame breaks down into methanol. When methanol is absorbed by the body, it converts to formaldehyde. Formaldehyde is embalming fluid. (Yes, that's in our food.) Formaldehyde can damage the immune and nervous systems. Start reading your labels—aspartame is in many of our foods and drinks. Try to locate a pack of gum that doesn't have aspartame in it. Side effects from aspartame can happen quickly, or it can build up over time. Many illnesses can be triggered or worsened by aspartame—multiple sclerosis, cancer, fibromyalgia, epilepsy, diabetes, chronic-fatigue syndrome, Parkinson's disease, and Alzheimer's disease. For the most updated information check out the Aspartame Consumer Safety Network.

Several books and studies have been written about its dangers:

* Consumption of Artificial Sweetener- and Sugar-containing Soda and Risk of Lymphoma and Leukemia in Men and Women. American Journal of Clinical Nutrition. Schernhammer, E. S., K. A. Bertrand, B. M. Birmann, L. Sampson, W. C. Willett, and D. Feskanich.
* Excitotoxins: The Taste That Kills. Russell L. Blaylock. Sante Fe, NM, Health, 1998.

Common foods with aspartame include sodas/pop, some juices and vegetable drinks, sweetened teas, flavored waters, some nutritional sports and energy drinks; hard candies; chewing gum; breath mints; yogurts;

ice creams; Popsicles; many sugar-free items like cookies, fruit spreads, maple syrups, ketchups; and even some over-the-counter medicines. It's important to avoid sugar-free or no-sugar-added products at all times, as they usually replace sugar with aspartame. It's very important to start reading your labels to see where aspartame is lurking in our foods.

Recently, the chemical companies began changing the name of aspartame on labels to "amino sweet," and yes, it's exactly the same toxin; it just has a new name to try to fool us.

The list below shows many of the side effects you may experience from aspartame.

Aspartame Toxicity Side Effects:

Numbness	Irritability	Aggression
Neuritis	Vertigo	Memory loss
Depression	Abdominal pain	Heart palpitations
Migraines	Anxiety	Weakness
Slurred speech	Weight gain	Asthma attacks
Nausea	Blurred vision	Skin allergies

Many of the symptoms from aspartame or amino-sweet toxicity mimic MS symptoms. I learned that if I consumed something containing aspartame, I would get an immediate headache and feel very "off" in my mind, as if I couldn't think properly or as if I had a sudden onset of brain fog.

Another very potent and dangerous GMO additive in our foods is MSG (monosodium glutamate). You are probably unknowingly eating MSG almost every day. It is the most widely used flavor enhancer because it's cheap to use and causes massive addiction because it makes food taste good. It will actually make you crave certain foods. MSG is used in processed foods, fast foods, Chinese foods, canned foods, and most frozen foods, and it's also widely used in restaurants.

The list below shows some common symptoms from eating MSG. Have you experienced any of these?

MSG Toxicity Side Effects:

Headaches	Diarrhea	Mood swings
Upset stomach	Skin rashes	Irritable bowel syndrome
Mental confusion	Arthritis	Behavioral problems (children)
Nausea	Dizziness	Heart palpitations
Vomiting	Depression	Anxiety/Panic attacks
Insomnia	Asthma attacks	Heart attack-like symptoms

Here is a list of names that manufacturers use in order to avoid disclosing that MSG is in our food. In my mind, it's just another way to deceive us.

Names in which MSG may be hidden:

<u>Hydrolyzed</u> vegetable protein	Barley Malt	Subu
<u>Natural</u> flavoring	Textured protein	Flavorings
<u>Hydrolyzed</u> milk protein	Calcium caseinate	Glutacyl
<u>Hydrolyzed</u> oat flavor	Gourmet powder	Spices (sometimes)
<u>Natural</u> beef flavoring	Sodium caseinate	Malt flavoring
<u>Hydrolyzed</u> plant protein	Seasonings	<u>Autolyzed</u> yeast
<u>Natural</u> pork flavoring	Gluteveve	Kombo extract

Notice that I've underlined the words "hydrolyzed," "autolyzed," and "natural"—those are key indicators that what you are consuming is actually MSG. It's quite shocking when you start to read labels and realize that these chemicals may be the key to our own health challenges. Yes, they are that dangerous to us.

The good news is that we know how to turn things around—just start eating healthy! Stay away from processed foods, eat more fruits and veggies, and definitely start reading your labels.

If you're putting chemical-laden foods into your body, you will definitely be affected in a negative way, and it can hurt your nervous system, your gut, and your immune system. Think about it: you're either eating to heal and help your body, or you're eating junk with additives and chemicals that can lead to disease, cancer, and maybe even death. I want you to remember that it's important to live your life and not to be so strict and rigorous with your food choices that you are miserable or that you make everyone else around you miserable. Think of this as a lifestyle and day by day make smart food choices for yourself.

Some people think they eat OK; they're pretty healthy, so they feel they can keep eating all these unhealthy foods and have no health issues, but just as water erodes a rock after time, horrible eating habits can erode your body and your good health.

CHAPTER 8

Nutritional Supplements

*"You can trace every sickness, every disease and every
ailment to a mineral [a nutrient] deficiency."*

—DR. LINUS PAULING

I BELIEVE NUTRITIONAL, WHOLE-FOOD SUPPLEMENTS are one of the most important items to add to your diet. It was life-changing for me. Many people change their diets to healthy ones only for a brief amount of time. Some people find it difficult to continue on this path long term, since it does take a huge commitment to change. I look at it as a lifestyle choice.

I know that for some, talking about supplements is very controversial. The school of thought seems to be that if you change your diet to organics and more clean eating, you'll no longer need supplements, but with our Western diet and our need for fast food and quick fixes, we need to add something every day that will be healthy, fast, and consistent. That's where nutritional supplements come into play. I know firsthand how beneficial they can be to MS sufferers. Adding supplements to my diet is the one thing I've done consistently for more than sixteen years. I know they have helped me control my MS, made me stronger, and helped combat chronic fatigue. They're an integral part of me living symptom-free.

Nutritional supplements can help strengthen your immune system, reduce inflammation, and provide antioxidants to fight free radicals that can run rampant through your body. They can help to heal your gut so you can absorb all the nutrients from your food. They will also help with fatigue and give you mental clarity. I supplement daily with an enzyme-based vitamin D-3 with K-2. I take an enzyme-based multivitamin and probiotics. I drink a vitamin-packed healthy energy drink high in B vitamins and other essential nutrients that has cured me of chronic fatigue. I drink a functional beverage with antioxidant and anti-inflammatory properties utilizing the muscadine grape. I also take Liposomal C.

One thing to make very clear is that supplementation will in no way compensate for your continued bad eating choices or unhealthy lifestyle. It won't. We have to change our eating habits to change our disease. We have to change our lifestyles to change our disease, and we have to change our thinking about everything related to MS and our long-term health!

Remember, with MS, you're not like everyone else. You have to find a balance in life, not only personally and professionally, but also with your nutrition if you're looking to be healthy, active, and have a better quality of life. This isn't a quick fix, it's a lifestyle.

VITAMIN D

I wish I could put this section's title in flashing lights! I would have confetti flying and music playing to show the importance of vitamin D. Perhaps one of the greatest discoveries relating to MS (and maybe to all autoimmune diseases, even cancer) is the benefits of the all-powerful vitamin D. Vitamin D can not only alleviate symptoms of MS and stop its progression, it can also prevent it. I have been eagerly following the Mayo Clinic and several European studies for many years, as they are on the forefront of the newest information related to MS and vitamin D.

Vitamin-D deficiency is a growing epidemic across the world and contributes largely to many debilitating diseases. Vitamin D can also help reduce the risk of common cancers, muscle and joint pains, and multiple sclerosis.

Isn't that incredible news? Can vitamin D actually prevent MS?

A simple blood test can tell you what your vitamin levels are. I've always asked my doctors to run my levels. Many doctors don't focus on vitamin levels and our overall health. Most MS sufferers and many people with autoimmune challenges have been shown to be very low in vitamin D. In some patients, vitamin D was almost nonexistent. Those may be the people who are suffering the worst MS symptoms and challenges. Some people experienced lower levels of vitamin D just before an exacerbation or even during an attack. It's interesting to note that in our society, we focus so much on staying out of the sun that we have an epidemic of vitamin D deficiency in people of all ages. We need to understand that modest sun exposure can be a great health benefit.

Here are some contributing factors to vitamin-D deficiency:

- A lack of sunny days
- A lack of oily fish in the diet
- Too much time indoors (it's estimated that Americans spend 90 percent of their time indoors)
- Covering the skin or using sunscreen on sunny days

- An inability to absorb vitamin D
  - People with heavy-metal toxicity will not be able to absorb it; I had this challenge
  - People on disease-modifying drugs may not be able to absorb it
  - People with celiac disease may not be able to absorb it

Vitamin-D deficiency causes these conditions:

- Multiple sclerosis
- Autism
- Heart disease
- Psoriasis
- Hypertension
- Cancer
- Depression
- Crohn's disease
- Eczema
- Asthma
- Obesity
- Rheumatoid arthritis
- TB
- Alzheimer's disease

The sun is the best source of vitamin D. That seems simple enough. The sun contributes significantly to the daily production of vitamin D in as little as fifteen to twenty minutes of exposure. In fact, that's thought to be enough time to prevent any deficiencies, but as any MS sufferer knows, each person is different, and you may not be able to get all your vitamin D that way. It's also hard to get consistent intake of vitamin D from foods.

Consistent sun exposure is difficult to do for those of us in northern climates. We know sun exposure can definitely increase vitamin D levels, and this may also be the reason MS is found at higher concentrations in countries and states that have less sunlight. In Illinois specifically, in the spring and summer months, I try to get myself and my family outside every morning for at least fifteen minutes wearing shorts and tanks (really, as little clothing as possible). Exposing your skin is very important. Living in Illinois, we cannot do that on a consistent basis throughout the year. We must look at alternatives to getting our vitamin D. We have turned to healthy supplements of vitamin D-3 with K-2 and light therapy. It's important to take your D-3 with K-2 as it supports the absorption and makes sure there's no calcification, which can actually harden your arteries.

The Mayo Clinic has a tremendous amount of information on vitamin D. You can go to their website and spend quite some time studying this single topic. I highly recommend becoming as knowledgeable as possible on this because of the overwhelming evidence showing us the benefits of vitamin D in preventing, treating, and even stopping the horrible effects of MS. The Mayo Clinic has many studies showing the different protocols of vitamin D therapy on MS sufferers. It's very intriguing info. If you go to their website and look at recommended dosages for vitamin D, there is a list for not only MS sufferers, but also for those suffering from many other chronic illnesses.

My doctors told me that it's extremely safe to supplement with vitamin D. For MS, the research indicates that it may be necessary to go on higher dosages so that levels are raised quickly in hopes of turning around the disease course. Also, one important point to make about your vitamin-D level is that the standards are different for disease prevention and treatment and what standardized medicine (non-holistic or functional medical practitioners) follow. I've had my vitamin-D levels tested many times, and my regular GP said my levels were normal— that is, there was no need to do anything different. My first response was, "Normal for whom? Normal for what condition?" My levels tested several times at less than 50 ng/ml, even less than 40 ng/ml. When I went to my holistic doctors with those same numbers, they immediately put me on a protocol of higher vitamin-D dosages of 20,000 IUs a day for several months to get my levels up. I always strive to get my levels from 70 to 100 ng/ml.

Always talk to your trusted healthcare provider about what supplements you should take and their recommended dosages. I'm not giving medical advice, only sharing what I've done.

What about Tanning Beds/UV Lights and Vitamin D?

Dr. Joseph Mercola is a world-renowned health professional, licensed physician, and surgeon in the state of Illinois. He's also a *New York Times* best-selling author; he has been featured on *The Today Show*, Dr. Oz, CNN, ABC's *World News Tonight*, CBS, NBC, and ABC's local news shows. Dr. Mercola does not recommend commercial tanning beds; he does, however, agree with healthy UVB light therapy. Go to Mercola.com, and look at his vitamin D resource page for the most comprehensive information on this nutrient and also benefits of light therapy.

Light therapy benefits include:

* Cardiovascular improvement
* Cancer prevention
* Skin repair
* Diabetes and osteoporosis prevention
* Bone and muscle support

Just recently, when I was at my dermatologist's office, I saw that he had a wall-mounted UVB light system. My doctor said he uses it to give a little vitamin D to patients who can't get out in the winter months and also to help treat those patients with SAD (seasonal affective disorder), which is a mood disorder or depression created by a lack of sunlight. He also stated that he has successfully been using this treatment for more than twenty-five years, and it has proved to be a great benefit to his patients.

I hope you can start your own research on vitamin D to understand its benefits and also to learn about the negative impact it can have on your whole body if you're deficient in this mineral.

I use vitamin D-3 supplements every day. I take 8,000 IU of vitamin D-3 during the winter months and 4,000 IU a day during the summer months when I'm able to get outside in the sun more often. I also use light therapy during the winter months. There is overwhelming evidence about the benefits of vitamin D and actually preventing and curing MS altogether.

(Support for the Vitamin D Hypothesis for Multiple Sclerosis Risk." *Nature Clinical Practice Neurology* 3.7 (2007): 358. Web.)

(Fitzgerald, Susan. "A New Genetic Study Associates Low Vitamin D and Risk for Multiple Sclerosis." *Neurology Today* 15.18 (2015): 1. Web.)

Important Herbs and Supplements

Coconut Oil and Coconut-Oil Supplements

Coconut oil is a powerful saturated fat with many benefits. Coconut-oil supplements can boost immunity; help fight illnesses, and aid digestion. Coconut oil contains important fatty acids that prevent illnesses. Some people won't take coconut oil because of the taste and prefer taking it in supplement form. Some believe that coconut oil is just another fad and that it can't really benefit us. Do your research. I know some people following specific MS diets that monitor fat intake who would not take coconut oil. I don't supplement or cook with coconut oil, I added it here because if you are researching any topics on healthy living, you will undoubtedly run into information on coconut oil. Many people believe it's a key ingredient to their healthy lifestyle.

PROBIOTICS

It seems everyone is talking about probiotics. It's the "it" word when talking about overall health. You break "probiotics" into two parts— "pro," meaning promoting, and "biotic," meaning life. I always think about probiotics as prolife and healthy bacteria. When we look at "antibiotics," the word means "antilife"; they kill bacteria.

It's important to have a healthy balance of bacteria in our gut because they filter out toxins. They also help our bodies to absorb the good things we need. Probiotics are known to help our immune systems function properly. Many holistic practitioners and doctors believe that the way to heal the entire body is by healing the gut. When you think about it logically, everything passes through our gut. Have you ever taken antibiotics? If so, then you needed to pump up on your probiotics to build up your immune system and start adding the good bacteria back into your body. When our immune systems aren't functioning properly, that's when we start to have autoimmune challenges like MS, Crohn's disease, rheumatoid arthritis, etc. I take a whole-food, enzyme-based probiotic. I also enjoy Kefir.

Probiotic rich foods: Kefir, sauerkraut, miso, kimchi, kombucha.

CALCIUM

Calcium has been known to help those with MS, in addition to its benefits of building strong bones and teeth. Calcium, along with vitamin D and even magnesium, may help repair nerve-tissue damage.

My multivitamin has calcium and magnesium. I also take another supplement that has calcium, magnesium, and potassium.

Calcium rich foods: Green leafy vegetables, kefir, broccoli, cheese, raw milk, almonds.

Vitamin B-1 (Thiamine)

Thiamine aids the nervous system in functioning properly. Lack of this nutrient can cause degeneration of the myelin sheath. Many MS symptoms can mimic this type of deficiency. The multivitamin and energy drink I take every day both have this important nutrient.

Vitamin B-1 rich foods: Green peas, spinach, asparagus, ground flaxseed, sunflower seeds.

Vitamin B-6

Vitamin B-6 ensures a healthy nervous system and immune system. Vitamin-B deficiencies can cause symptoms of anemia, chronic fatigue, and even confusion. This is also in my healthy energy drink and my multivitamin.

Vitamin B-6 rich foods: Wild caught salmon or tuna, banana, grass-fed beef, sweet potato, spinach.

Vitamin B-12

Vitamin B-12 is an essential nutrient for neurological function and is vitally important to an MS sufferer because it is needed to help develop nerve cells. The myelin sheath coating our nerves cannot successfully form if there is a vitamin B-12 deficiency. In fact, this is another vitamin deficiency that will give us symptoms similar to our MS symptoms.

Vitamin B-12 injections are very popular for people with MS and other health conditions.

Vitamin B-12 rich foods: Sardines, wild caught salmon or tuna, grass-fed beef, raw milk or cheese.

VITAMIN A
Vitamin A plays a role in maintaining healthy vision, bone growth, cell reproduction, and cell strength. Vitamin A plays a huge role in keeping our immune systems strong. I take a healthy, vitamin-packed energy drink each day that has vitamin A and plenty of the all-important B vitamins.

Vitamin A rich foods: Carrots, sweet potato, kale, spinach, romaine lettuce, cantaloupe.

VITAMIN C
Vitamin C helps in building collagen. Vitamin C is, of course, great for fighting off a cold, but it also protects our bodies from stress, lowers cholesterol, and many people use it while dealing with cancer or to prevent cancer. I take 1,000 to 2,000 IU of Liposomal C each day.

Vitamin C rich foods: Oranges, kale, green and red peppers, strawberries, broccoli.

COENZYME Q_{10} (CoQ_{10})
Coenzyme Q_{10} is a naturally occurring enzyme in the body that helps with cell function. It has been shown to reduce inflammation and boost our immune system's function. It will also help improve MS sufferers' fatigue. My doctor recommended that I take a supplement form as food sources have such low levels of this nutrient.

CoQ$_{10}$ rich foods: Grass fed beef, organic chicken, broccoli, strawberries, oranges, sesame seeds.

VITAMIN E
Vitamin E helps protect cells from the damage caused by free radicals. It's also needed for a healthy immune system and nervous system. Vitamin-E deficiency can cause challenges with coordination and brain function. Vitamin E is another component in my healthy energy drink and multivitamin.

Vitamin E rich foods: Sunflower seeds, mango, almonds, hazelnuts, broccoli.

L-CARNITINE
L-Carnitine is great at reducing fatigue, increasing energy, and protecting muscles, and it can also boost cognition. I take this every day as well. It's another ingredient in the energy drink I have every morning. I believe this is one of the key items that helped me cure my chronic-fatigue syndrome.

L-Carnitine rich foods: Grass-fed beef, organic chicken, asparagus.

FOLATE AND FOLIC ACID
Folate is another B vitamin that has a slightly different function from the others. It is found naturally in foods, while folic acid is the synthetic form usually found in supplements. It helps new cells grow and helps old cells repair themselves, and it will help maintain nerve function.

Folate rich foods: Garbanzo beans, lentils, asparagus, beets, broccoli.

GINSENG
Ginseng is a wonderful anti-inflammatory herb. It can help reduce stress, fatigue, and depression, and it can even help maintain mental clarity. I take this every day. Many people enjoy this in tea.

VITAMIN K-2
Vitamin K is just as important for our bodies as vitamin D. Vitamin K helps with blood clotting, prevents heart disease, and builds strong bones. Vitamin K decreases inflammation and helps us process vitamin D. Vitamin K-2 is in my vitamin D-3 supplement and my multivitamin.

Vitamin K rich foods: Kale, Brussel sprouts, cabbage, cucumbers, broccoli.

MAGNESIUM
Magnesium is an essential nutrient to support our nervous system. Magnesium deficiency can also cause symptoms comparable to our MS symptoms—depression, mental fogginess, tremors, numbness, and tingling. I take this every day.

Magnesium rich foods: Spinach, pumpkin seeds, almonds, chard, avocado.

OMEGA-3
Omega-3 fatty acids help our immune systems and neurological functions. They promote cardiovascular health and even improve brain function. This is one of those supplements that seem to be getting a lot of attention now. It's found in fish oils and in flaxseed oil. The Overcoming Multiple Sclerosis Diet recommends people with MS get their omega-3s from flaxseed oil rather than fish oil.

Omega-3 rich foods: Walnuts, chia seeds, wild caught salmon and tuna, flaxseed.

ZINC

Your immune system needs zinc to defend itself effectively against viruses. My supplements also have zinc in them. I do have a supplement that is high in zinc that I take if I feel a cold coming on, or if I'm around people who are ill. I think of it as my cold-and-virus protector.

Zinc rich foods: Grass fed beef, garbanzo beans, pumpkin seeds, cashews.

TURMERIC (CURCUMIN)

Turmeric has been used for thousands of years, and the most up-to-date research shows that its medicinal qualities can help your whole body. Turmeric is a natural anti-inflammatory and can help the immune system. In a Vanderbilt medical study, it blocked the progression of MS in mice. In countries where turmeric is part of the daily diet, MS is a very rare disease. Many people cook with turmeric, add it to their juices or smoothies, and even drink turmeric tea.

(Natarajan C, Bright JJ. Paper presented at the Annual Experimental Biology 2002 Conference New Orleans, LA April 23, 2002.)

GINGER

Ginger is another spice, like turmeric, that has anti-inflammatory properties and can support immune function. Ginger can give relief from infections, muscle and joint pain, nausea, indigestion, headache, cardiovascular disease, and it can protect against cancer and even help mental clarity. Many people cook with ginger and use it in juicing. My family loves ginger, and it is a staple in our house for all of our daily juicing. It's a key component in my supplements. I also use ginger when I travel, for motion sickness and to help my immune system.

My Thoughts about Supplements and Herbs
There is so much groundbreaking information on supplements and herbs and their overall benefit to our bodies that it's worth thoroughly investigating. Supplements and herbs can help keep your immune system strong. I know this is the one thing I have done consistently throughout the past sixteen years, and I feel 100 percent better because of it. You'll want to speak with your nutritionist or health-care provider about what supplement and herb protocol they would recommend.

CHAPTER 9

Creating the Best Body

ALTHOUGH I DON'T USE DRUG therapy for treatment of my MS, and I haven't since 1999, I know plenty of people do. With what I now personally know about MS, I cannot recommend drug therapy to anyone. The side effects and long-term effects on our bodies are far too serious and should never be taken lightly.

I'm of the opinion that we need to look at treating the whole body to become healthy and strong and beat MS. You'll hear me state my mantra over and over: "A healthy immune system equals a healthy body." Having a properly functioning immune system is the first step to lifelong health.

On the journey with MS, we must realize that just as there wasn't one thing that made us sick, there isn't just one thing that will heal us. It is a culmination of many things. We need to focus on what we eat, what we absorb, what we breathe in, what supplements we take, our activity level, our mind-set, and how our relationships function.

With MS, there are many things we can do to optimize our health, stay strong physically and mentally, and repair the damage this disease has done to our bodies. The next area I want to cover is what we need to do to create the best body, and what the medical community deems complementary and alternative medicine (CAM). These are practical steps and treatments you can take to deal with your body as a whole, so you can become renewed, healthy, and strong. The most common reason for using CAMs is the desire to use holistic healthcare that recognizes the interrelatedness of mind, body, and spirit. I looked to these alternatives because of my own frustration with conventional medicine. I have to share that I didn't know what I didn't know; do you ever think about that saying? If I hadn't been told there was a different way, I would still be following traditional protocols. The truth is that when I followed the standard advice from my doctors and used the traditional MS fixes, I was really sick; I kept having flare-ups, exacerbations, and I had a horrible quality of life. They wanted me to follow the standard MS protocol of drug therapy: take one type of disease-modifying drug to start, then a drug for pain, then a drug for depression, and so on. It was a slippery slope to a medicine cabinet full of garbage that wasn't doing any good. This traditional approach was hurting my body, not restoring it.

WE NEED TO STAY PROACTIVE ABOUT OUR HEALTH

When I decided I would no longer go the traditional medical route for treating my MS, I started searching for things that could help create and support the healthy body I needed. I focused on ways to help me de-stress, repair, energize, align, and balance - approaches that would make me stronger physically and mentally. What I found restored my health and vitality. I believe these things saved my life!

It's also important to note that all the information I'm sharing has been around for many years, some of it for thousands of years. If only I had known.

MASSAGE

I am hooked on massage; it was a catalyst in my recovery, and I know it continues to repair my body.

Here are the most common types of massage:

- Swedish massage is a gentle form of massage that uses long strokes, kneading, deep circular movements, and tapping to help relax and energize you. (I prefer Swedish massage; I find it to be the most relaxing.)
- Deep-tissue massage uses slower, more forceful strokes to target the deeper layers of muscle. (I have always hated deep-tissue massage; I'm all about relaxation. My best friend loves her deep-tissue massages, to me, they're pure torture.)
- Sports massage is similar to Swedish massage, but it is geared toward people involved in sporting activities. It can be used to help prevent or treat injuries. Many people use it to prepare themselves for sporting events.
- The raindrop technique is something I recently learned about when talking to my massage therapist. It seems very promising. It was developed by Gary Young, the founder of Young Living Essential Oils. It is an application of highly antimicrobial essential oils directly to the spine with effleurage (finger-stroking) techniques to distribute healing energy throughout the body. This technique has been praised highly by users all over the world for its help with relaxation, emotional release, tissue cleansing, and spinal misalignments. The use of essential oils such as peppermint, frankincense, and sandalwood can potentially be very successful in treating or minimizing the symptoms of multiple sclerosis or other neurodegenerative diseases, depression, and dementia.

BENEFITS OF REGULAR MASSAGE

PHYSICAL BENEFITS:

- Relaxes the body
- Calms the nervous system
- Lowers blood pressure
- Slows respiration
- Reduces chronic pain
- Loosens tight muscles
- Improves skin tone
- Reduces swelling
- Improves posture
- Improves muscle tone
- Reduces tension headaches
- Increases tissue metabolism
- Decreases muscle deterioration
- Increases range of motion
- Speeds elimination of metabolic waste
- Increases blood and lymph circulation
- Increases red blood cell count
- Strengthens the immune system
- Improves skin tone
- Speeds recovery from injury

MENTAL BENEFITS:

- Reduces stress
- Promotes quality sleep
- Improves productivity
- Induces mental relaxation
- Improves concentration

EMOTIONAL BENEFITS:

- Reduces anxiety
- Enhances self-image
- Provides a sense of well-being
- Nurtures emotional growth

I recommend getting a massage at least twice a month. I noticed benefits from massage right away, and its effects will be something that stays with you. Remember, this journey is about healing, repairing, and restoring our bodies.

Much of the information in this section is shared from Massage Envy, The MS Society, and from other massage therapists that I've worked with.

CHIROPRACTIC CARE

I started using chiropractic care back in 1998 after I was in a car accident in which I sustained horrible whiplash. My neck bothered me periodically because of the trauma of that accident and my poor posture. When I started doing research on MS and alternative treatments, I learned how chiropractic care worked and how it could help my body be in alignment.

When I learned that misalignment of the spine is often associated with trauma—car accidents, sports injuries, slips and falls, bad sleeping habits, incorrect lifting, and even poor posture (which I had), it made sense for me to go check it out.

Generally speaking, chiropractic care is the use of conservative methods that include hands-on therapies that affect the body's unique ability to heal itself. Chiropractic care is proactive, not reactive. It focuses on prevention rather than intervention. This statement alone is a core difference between chiropractic and traditional medical care. We all need to be proactive with our health.

I was sold on the benefits of chiropractic care after my first visit. I felt less pain in my neck and back and even felt refreshed. So when I started looking at it for helping my MS, it made perfect sense that it could be of great help in healing my body.

I love chiropractic care because it helps your body without the use of drugs. It's all about aligning the neck and spine for optimal health and increased immune-system function. Since a healthy immune system is necessary to combat MS, it seemed simple enough to understand how this could be a huge benefit.

Some benefits of chiropractic care include:

* Pain management
* Lower blood pressure
* Increased range of movement
* Increased immune-system function
* Reduced pain from headaches or migraines
* Improved sleep quality
* Improved nervous-system function

My family and I now use chiropractic care consistently as a preventative and maintenance measure.

ACUPUNCTURE

As described by the MS Society, acupuncture is one form of traditional Chinese medicine. It's based on a theory about body functioning that involves the flow of energy known as *qi* ("chee") through fourteen pathways called meridians throughout the body. Acupuncture involves stimulating specific locations on the skin, usually by inserting thin, disposable metallic needles into points along the meridians in the body in order to alter the flow of energy. According to the theories of Chinese medicine, disease results from an imbalance or disruption in the flow of energy between the opposing forces of *yin* and *yang*.

I looked into acupuncture while I was receiving chiropractic care, and I learned that acupuncture can stimulate the immune system. As you've heard me say repeatedly throughout this book, it's important to have a healthy immune system. And doesn't it make sense to do anything and everything possible to try to have a healthy, properly functioning immune system? Now, my MS doctors always told me to avoid chiropractic care, acupuncture, and even supplements; they said those would stimulate my immune system. If I had followed their tactics, I would still be sick and relapsing. Certain things make sense, and doing everything to repair the immune system is what I started to focus on. I've always believed that once your immune system is healthy and functioning properly, it's healed.

According to the National MS Society, many MS sufferers use acupuncture for the relief of pain, muscle spasms, numbness, tingling, fatigue, depression, anxiety, and bowel and bladder symptoms.

The benefits of acupuncture are amazing, and that is the one thing I turned to in the beginning of my journey to start the process of healing. I did acupuncture for many years to help my body get into alignment and in sync, and I use it today to keep my body that way. I believe acupuncture helps your mind, body, and spirit through each course of treatment.

MEDITATION

I started meditating about six years ago; it was something very new to me. One of my good friends, Mayra, loaned me a book called *The Monk Who Sold His Ferrari* by Robin Sharma, a successful leadership teacher, coach, and the bestselling author of fifteen books. You can find out all about him at RobinSharma.com. This was a life-changing book for me in many ways, and I was kind of obsessed with it. On top of the many Post-its and highlights Mayra put in, I also read it, reread it, and then read it again, adding my own squiggles, highlights, and tabs. Mayra was gracious enough to let me keep her copy, and I highly recommend you get this book too. There's a chapter in the book that teaches about beginning meditation with the Heart of the Rose technique. (You'll need a rose for this) It's all about calming your mind and having no other thoughts besides the rose. It taught me how to focus on the petals, colors, smells, stem, and thorns; it was definitely challenging at first, but it can be done. You really can quiet your mind to outside distractions or thoughts.

I know what you may be thinking. *There is so much going on—too many things to do and many challenges and issues to deal with—how can I possibly quiet my mind?* I totally understand. I had challenges meditating at first too. However, if you're serious about learning a great technique for beginning your meditation, and improving your health in the long run, you will definitely want to check this out. From the first time I started to meditate, no matter where I was and no matter what state of mind I was in, it made me feel better. I felt a sense of calm. I felt strong, focused, centered, and at peace.

If you meditate, you know exactly what I mean. For those of you who have not meditated and are suffering from MS, another autoimmune disease, or the many stresses of life itself, meditation could be the one thing that acts as a vehicle to make you stronger, calmer, more centered, and more peaceful.

> "Your body is precious. It is our vehicle for awakening.
> Treat it with care."
>
> —BUDDHA

Meditation is very popular now. Some people focus on it for spiritual awakening, while others simply use it as a tool for stress reduction, relaxation, and self-improvement. I have been a student for many of the past sixteen years focusing on health, nutrition, personal growth, spirituality, leadership, success, and relationships. It's so important to grow as a person and to learn new things, especially when you have MS; it will help your brain stay sharp. That has always been important to me. In fact, instead of having a big party for my fortieth birthday, I went with my girlfriends Tammy and Mayra to a special event with

Jack Canfield, America's #1 success coach, the founder of the billion-dollar book brand *Chicken Soup for the Soul*, and a leading authority on peak performance and life success. The training we attended was called "Breakthrough to Success." This training focused specifically on his *New York Times* best-selling book called *The Success Principles*, a life-changing book I highly recommend. In that training, Jack taught many key points that actually helped me deal with not only life, but also with this disease. Jack also taught us how important meditation is because it can help you access your intuition, solve problems, achieve goals, and calm yourself from the inside out. I believe it can change your entire life.

Jack taught us that as you meditate, you'll become more spiritually attuned. You'll be able to better discern and even recognize the sound of your higher self or the voice of God speaking to you through words, images, and sensations. Yes, it's that powerful!

At that event, we heard how some people had amazing breakthroughs, experiences, and transformations by meditating. In fact, through the guided meditations we had that week, I experienced clarity, focus, and an amazing sense of calm that permeated my whole body. I learned that you can get that feeling every time you meditate.

As any MS sufferer knows, the mind is incredibly powerful. It's so powerful, that patients will sometimes start to manifest symptoms they have read about or discussed with others. When you meditate, you can manifest positive, uplifting thoughts that will help you.

Meditation will calm and quiet your mind. It can reduce stress, give you a better perspective when dealing with stressful situations, improve sleep, lower blood pressure, help with pain, fight fatigue, lessen depression, stop anxiety, enhance mental clarity, and overall, it can strengthen your immune system. You can meditate in a quiet space, with music or chanting, or even by listening to a guided meditation.

TYPES OF MEDITATION:

* Mantra Meditation – Repeat a calming word or phrase
* Yoga – Perform a series of poses with controlled breathing exercises
* Tai Chi – While deep breathing you perform a series of movements
* Qi Gong – Meditation combined with relaxation, movement and breathing
* Guided Meditation – Sometimes called visualization – usually led by a teacher. You form mental images you find relaxing, or what the teacher talks about.
* Transcendental Meditation – This technique is used by Dr. Oz. Using a word, sound, or phrase repeatedly and silently to calm your mind and think of nothing else.

> "All that we are is the result of what we have thought.
> The mind is everything. What we think we become."
>
> —BUDDHA

PILATES

Exercise not only improves your overall health and well-being, it also helps manage many MS symptoms, and Pilates is one form of therapeutic exercise. The Pilates Method was created during World War I by Joseph H. Pilates, a German inventor, boxer, and dancer. He developed the technique to help soldiers recover from war injuries. Pilates is extremely popular, especially with MS sufferers.

Pilates is a method where individuals concentrate on body movements. There are more than five hundred movements that focus on very specific muscles and how they are controlled. There also is an emphasis on deep, coordinated breathing. These breathing techniques are wonderful to help center you during workouts.

I absolutely *love* Pilates. You can see benefits from Pilates immediately. It strengthens your muscles and supports your core. If you have a strong core, it will help support your back and legs.

I believe the Pilates Reformer machine gave me maximum health benefits without strain or stress on my body. There are many pieces of Pilates equipment that provide gravity-based resistance training. I use the Pilates Reformer because even though I am not very flexible or coordinated, it improved my core muscles, strengthened my other muscles, and helped me become more limber without a lot of impact on my body.

You can also use a floor mat to do Pilates. That was more challenging for me because I was so inflexible. A good Pilates instructor can provide an assessment and find the right workout for you. There are plenty of Pilates instructors who have specific workout plans for those with MS.

Yoga

Yoga is an ancient practice that combines poses, breathing techniques, and meditation to connect body, mind, and spirit to increase your strength and flexibility. Some people find that yoga improves their energy levels and their moods. Yoga can be adapted to the needs and abilities of someone living with MS. Even though yoga is often listed as a type of meditation, it has other far-reaching health benefits:

- Relieves chronic pain
- Reduces fatigue
- Relieves depression and anxiety

* Improves muscle spasticity
* Helps overcome joint stiffness
* Increases oxygen in the blood
* Promotes relaxation
* Improves sleep quality
* Boosts the immune system
* Stimulates the lymphatic system

I have tried yoga several times throughout the years, and I have to say it wasn't my favorite. I was inflexible, so it was very painful. I have several friends who sing yoga's praises for helping them with pain, improving their flexibility, and also providing them with a great sense of peace and calm. I recommend trying several activities to see what you enjoy the most. You should seek out yoga instructors who have specific knowledge of MS symptoms; they can devise a workout best suited for you.

WEIGHTLIFTING AND STRENGTH TRAINING

I've worked out all my life. I was in sports throughout school and even bought a gym membership when I was sixteen. One important thing to understand is that a lack of physical activity can weaken your muscles, deteriorate your bones, increase your risk of heart disease, lead to depression, and increase fatigue. Strong muscles are more capable of withstanding stress.

Weightlifting can improve muscle strength, reduce fatigue, improve your range of motion, prevent osteoporosis, and help you get motivated. Personally, I love lifting weights. If you're new to lifting weights, you can go to a gym or you can work out at home. To help keep you on track, I recommend lifting with a friend or loved one. When you lift weights or do strength training, you automatically start to feel stronger. It's very empowering.

You can use weight machines or free weights. Even if you have limited mobility, there are weights to work out just about any part of your body, so you can still reap some benefits. When you work out, make sure to drink plenty of water to keep yourself hydrated, and make sure you are not getting overheated.

WATER THERAPY

Water therapy/exercise may be the easiest and lowest-impact way for someone with MS to stay active. According to the National MS Society, it can strengthen and relax muscles, help your balance, improve flexibility, reduce pain, and lessen stress. I don't use water therapy, but I wanted to add this because no matter what physical issues you may be having now, water therapy can be tailored to your exact needs.

WORKING OUT WITH TRAINERS

If you do work out with a trainer, it's important to make sure he or she understands your physical condition now and your MS. For many years, I went to see trainers or even physical therapists who overworked me with lots of cardio, either riding a bike or walking on a treadmill, and that was too much. They didn't understand that if we weren't already experiencing numbness or tingling in our legs, and we over did it with these types of activities, we could automatically start to feel pain, numbness, tingling, and in some cases, there may be temporary loss of mobility in our legs and feet. Over the years, I learned that if I was having any problems with numbness or tingling in my legs, I needed to stay away from that type of cardio altogether. However, once I started lifting weights, I never worried about the cardio because you're definitely working out your heart when you lift weights.

Whatever way you choose to make your best body from the information I shared above, make sure to have fun, listen to your body, and focus on continued improvement day by day to ensure your health and happiness.

Before you start any type of exercise program, speak to your trusted healthcare provider.

CHAPTER 10

Give Me a Little More Attitude!

"The only difference between a good day
and a bad day is your attitude."

—Dennis S. Brown

WHAT IF I TOLD YOU that having a great attitude could greatly improve your MS? Some people may think that is a ridiculous statement. How could having a positive attitude or thinking positively help your health? Some of you may be thinking that this insight is a given. Either way, Attitude is an important topic, and it's at the ground level for becoming a healthier person. The health benefits of positive thinking and having a good attitude have been proven over and over again, in study after study.

In fact, being positive and having the right attitude can:

- Lower depression rates
- Increase life spans
- Strengthen immune system
- Reduce risks of heart conditions
- Reduce stress hormones
- Improve quality of sleep

Do you consider yourself pessimistic or optimistic? What about the all too familiar saying: Is your glass half empty or half full? I know you've heard this a million times, right? That conjures up different images in our minds. Your answer will determine if you have a scarcity or an abundance mentality.

Having a positive attitude does not mean you aren't fully aware of the circumstances and challenges surrounding you. Yes, we all have challenges; this is life, whether you are living with MS or not. Being positive simply means that you approach these instances with a more productive outlook. You are actually expecting good things to come to you, no matter what. When you choose to respond in a more positive way in a difficult situation, you are choosing not to be a victim of reactionary behavior.

Isn't it easy to be reactionary when something just pops up, takes you off course, or challenges you? Sometimes it's easy to lose control in a situation, right? We all have a hundred thoughts running through our heads every minute, both positive and negative. All of these thoughts affect our outlook on life. If we consistently work on thinking positive thoughts, we actually train our minds to be more optimistic and hopeful. If we are worried all the time and think negative thoughts, we train our minds to be negative and pessimistic.

This has been one of my greatest challenges. But when I slow down in a gritty situation and think about what I want my end result to be, it helps to demagnify an issue and helps me think in a more positive way. We've all been there. Someone cut you off while driving, was rude or short-tempered with you, or worse. What about dealing with someone who always has to be right? Have any of these situations happened to you? Let me also ask, what are you expecting to happen to you?

If you are expecting negative things to continue to happen to you (bad health, bad doctor visits, lack of support from friends or family, etc.), I guarantee you are going to continue experiencing that negative outcome.

Have you ever noticed how things can spiral out of control when something negative happens? Here's an example. What happens when you wake up in the morning only to realize the alarm didn't go off? You panic, right? You jump out of bed, stub your toe, and run around like crazy trying to find the match to your shoe, only to realize the dog has chewed it up. At this point, you are a raving lunatic who is yelling at the dog! You then jump in the car and realize you never filled up the gas tank. Next, you're stuck in rush-hour traffic and know you're going to be incredibly late for work. You get the picture: the day is going horribly wrong, and it is only getting worse as one bad thing happens after another for the entire day. Since you now have a bad attitude, you expect that more bad things will happen, and the rest of your day is shot.

Have you ever been in a situation like that? Did you wonder why things were going awry? Well, it was because you were in a negative state of mind, expecting negative things. And guess what? That's exactly what you'll get, every single time, over and over again. Negative attitudes perpetuate negative results. What you think about you bring about.

"Attitude is a little thing that makes a big difference."

—WINSTON CHURCHILL

I don't know about you, but for me, this was a real eye-opener. Things like this have happened to me, and maybe they've happened to you. What can we do to stop this madness? First, you can slow down. Take a deep breath, assess the situation, and decide what you actually want the end result to be. If you keep going in the above scenario, it will be pure madness for the rest of the day.

What transpired was already bad enough. You're upset, the poor dog will probably avoid you, you may have some penalty for being late for work, and now, you're going on with your day frustrated and angry. Whatever way you look at it, it does not pay to be reactionary. In this case, your horrible attitude, anger, and negativity will do more harm than good, not only to people you are dealing with, but to your own health as well.

What if you stopped and took a deep breath? What if you instead determined that you wanted your end result to be a good, positive, and productive day? How could you be more open minded in a stressful situation? What if you just stopped and laughed when you realized what had happened? What if you chalked it up to life? You could also make sure that you learn from this—so that there isn't a next time. There are many different ways to spin the situation; you can do it in a more positive and productive way, wouldn't you agree?

I challenge you to do a test that I've done in past stressful situations, when things went wrong, circumstances were out of my control, or when I had a confrontation with someone. Notice what starts to happen in your body; it's amazing how our bodies react. I felt my heart start to race, I started to get anxious, my head started to pound, and I could feel my stomach start to turn. Trust me, those feelings are not healthy. You need to listen to your body. Those feelings can lead to all kinds of health issues for you as they create increased levels of stress hormones and make your body acidic.

Now let's look at another scenario. Do you know any of those people who seem to go through life with positive attitudes, no matter what the circumstances? I do, and to be honest, it was irritating at times. I thought they weren't dealing with reality or that they just didn't get it. *Life is tough!* I thought. *Things are challenging! There's no one who can be that positive all the time.*

As I've grown, thank God, I've gained some wisdom and perspective. I've learned about the importance of having a good attitude, living in the moment, and being grateful for all I have. I realized that even though I didn't get it at the time, those positive people were on to something.

Imagine an uncomplicated life, one that is not overrun with negativity, doubt, and discouragement. Imagine expecting great things every day, responding to challenges in appropriate ways, dealing with issues—*and then letting them go.* I know you might be thinking that's easier said than done, is it? I've lived in both of the extremes—positive and negative—and the latter is detrimental to your health, to your relationships, and to your entire life.

How do you start on a path to thinking more positively? First, don't watch negative TV or the news and bypass that kind of stuff on social media. Think about it: people love to share the worst things that are going on in this world! If there is positive news, you usually have to sift through mounds of sad, negative, and depressing information to find it. That's unacceptable. Why is that the standard? Start looking at a negative situation and decide how you can turn it around to be positive.

I started learning about personal growth and healthy thinking many years ago, and I continue to learn tips and techniques today. They help me with my personal life, my spiritual life, and even my professional life. Here are some things you can do to help improve your attitude day by day. Remember, it's a process. No one is perfect, but by taking these actions, you'll learn to cope with issues as they arise in a healthier, more positive, and increasingly productive way.

Make a Gratitude Journal

Appreciation and gratitude are some of the highest emotional states you can be in, so it's important to try to incorporate both into your daily life. I write in my gratitude journal each night before bed; it's a great time to evaluate and reflect on the day, and writing it out puts everything in perspective.

Try this at bedtime tonight: grab some paper and a pen, and write down three or four things for which you are grateful. You'll see that thoughts start coming to you easily. Here's an example of what you can write in your journal:

* I am happy and grateful for having such a productive and stress-free day
* I am happy and grateful for feeling healthy and strong
* I am grateful for my family's support, love and encouragement
* I am grateful for my friends
* I am grateful for my dogs; they bring me joy and happiness
* I am grateful that I am able to help others

There is such power in gratitude. When we have an attitude of gratitude, great things will come to us.

I also like to look through my gratitude journal regularly, as it reminds me of just how truly blessed I am. In fact, it always puts a smile on my face. When you express gratefulness, your body cannot be in a state of sadness, depression, or negativity—the mind doesn't work like that.

I know some people will find that cultivating an attitude of gratitude and genuine appreciation requires a lot of change and diligence. We are taught early on in life to focus on the things we *don't* have. Instead, we should be taught to appreciate everything we have already received and to be happy where we are in that moment.

While studying under Jack Canfield, another great technique I learned from his *New York Times* best-selling book *The Success Principles* was how to create affirmations. "An affirmation is a statement that describes a goal in its already completed state." Affirmations are something you write about yourself and your life; just start by using "I am."

Here are some examples of positive affirmations:

- I am happily helping people with MS each and every day
- I love my renewed and healthy body
- I am excited and happy to be a best-selling author, speaker, coach,
- I am healthy, strong, and revitalized
- I am successful
- I am peaceful
- I am blessed
- I am grateful

You'll want to make short, concise statements. You'll notice I don't use negative words or phrases. How could the following statements be made more powerful?

- I am trying to be peaceful - *change to:* I am at peace
- I want to lose weight - *change to:* I am enjoying my ideal weight of...
- I need to pay off my debt - *change to:* I have more than enough money

These each have negative words (try, want, need, etc). In our minds, this comes back as lack, neediness, and negativity, which is not at all what an affirmation should conjure up in our minds.

When I do my affirmations, the thoughts and feelings that come to me are those of abundance, positivity, and strength. I know I am attracting more of what I want in my life, not empowering more of what I don't want.

Affirmations are something you can start doing right away. They are a great technique that will help you to change that negative self-talk we all tend to have in our heads. We all know we are our own worst critics. When you are feeling down, you can easily grab your gratitude journal or your affirmation journal and go through it to remind you of your blessings.

Yes, our mind, body, and spirits are connected. Studies have shown that people with positive attitudes heal more quickly from illnesses than people with negative attitudes.

One last tip—and this is a big deal—as you are working on that positive attitude, ask yourself a few questions about the people you spend time with:

* Are they pessimistic or optimistic?
* Do they make you laugh?
* Do they have good attitudes?
* Do they have positive energy?
* Are they supportive of you (whether they agree with you or not)?
* Do they accept you for who you are, faults and all?
* Are they there for you when you need them?
* Do they try to change you?
* Do they make you feel bad about your decisions?
* Do they try to manipulate you?
* Do they only care about themselves and their needs, instead of you and your needs?

You see, attitudes are catchy, whether they are positive or negative; either way, they are undoubtedly having an effect on you. And yes, they *will* rub off on you.

Make a list of the people you spend your time with, and look at those questions. Where do they fit in? The people around you will affect every aspect of your life, especially your health. If the people in your life are supportive and positive, that's great; you need them in your life. If the people in your life are pessimistic and negative, then you need to set up boundaries with them. (Yes, this might even be a family member.) Can you limit your contact with them? Make sure you set up guidelines so that you don't see each other so much. Don't spend time with people who drain your energy. Give it a try. It can work.

You can make conscious efforts every day to have a better attitude. I know for sure that this is something that can help your MS, and it can help every aspect of your life as it has helped mine.

Having the right attitude is a choice, and it's one you need to make to live a better, healthier, and more fulfilled life. So, it's OK to give everyone an attitude; just make sure it's a positive one!

(B. L. Fredrickson, "What Good Are Positive Emotions?", *Review of General Psychology,* no. 2 (1998): 300–319.)

CHAPTER 11

Laughter: Is It Really the Best Medicine?

WHILE WRITING THIS BOOK AND being in a healthy-living business, I've been voracious about studying health and nutrition, collecting information and statistics, talking with other MS sufferers, doctors, and holistic practitioners to find out everything I could about health, healing, and specifically, my MS. So in the spirit of research for this book, I decided to start asking the people closest to me some questions about what they thought were the contributing factors to why I'm doing so well.

I got a lot of different answers, and most touched on qualities such as being active, exercising, positive thinking, having a great attitude, and being a goofball, but there was one overarching theme—they all thought I laughed a lot.

When I looked back over the years, I realized that it's true. I am always laughing. I am always joking around, and I'm always looking at situations and making funny, smarty-pants comments about things. I don't know why I started doing that; maybe it's because I grew up in a stressful household with an overbearing dad and lots of siblings. Who knows, but I know that laughter can definitely defuse a sticky situation.

I believe laughter is another powerful way we can support a healthy immune system, fight disease, and live with a great quality of life. Our mind, body, and spirits are connected; therefore, healing in all those areas is necessary.

The focus on the benefits of laughter really began with Norman Cousins's memoir, *Anatomy of an Illness*. Cousins was diagnosed with ankylosing spondylitis, a painful spinal condition. He was bedridden and found that watching comedies like Marx Brothers films and episodes of *Candid Camera* helped him feel better. He stated that ten minutes of laughter allowed him two hours of pain-free sleep. Some hospitals around the country have incorporated laughter therapy into their protocols now.

In fact, there is research and data showing the health benefits of laughter. Two studies from the American College of Sports Medicine's 56th Annual Meeting in Seattle, 2009, found that laughter can not only reduce stress (which can damage the heart), it can also lead to improved blood flow, which can help ward off high blood pressure and heart disease. One test group watched a comedy, and the positive health effects lasted a full twenty-four hours after they watched it. It's also interesting to note that another test group watched a documentary on a depressing subject, and they had negative health effects.

Think about how infectious laughter is—one person starts laughing, then another, and then another. Laughter keeps people together; it boosts energy levels, attracts people to you, reduces pain, protects you from negativity and stress, and actually strengthens your immune system. It's that powerful. I've always believed it's important to laugh, be a goofball, and have fun.

Laughter can:

* Help your heart by increasing blood flow

* Give you pain relief
* Boost your immune system
* Help fight disease
* Reduce stress hormones levels (which suppress our immune systems)
* Most definitely relax your whole body
* Brighten your outlook on life

Laughter is a positive ingredient for your overall health, and it's important to laugh every day.

There is an urban legend stating that children laugh around four hundred times a day, while adults only laugh about twenty-five times a day. There is no scientific proof for this. However, somehow it makes sense that children laugh more. After all, they're kids; they should be playing, laughing, and goofing off as much as possible. Some adults may laugh more than others; you can check yourself on this. Do you laugh? Do you laugh often? Do you understand how laughter can impact your health?

As I think back about the past sixteen years of my life and my progression of being healthier, these benefits ring true for me. All I can say is that in that short amount of time, I have had what I would call a lifetime of silly experiences, situations, and memories.

Laughter is very cathartic. It can also help with disagreements and disappointments in most situations. In life, it's all about having the right perspective.

I really never cared about making other people laugh at my expense; I basically laugh along. As I've grown as a person, it's interesting how I've attracted certain people into my life. The friends I have in my life are here for a reason, and I can laugh with them about anything. I can be silly or dorky or whatever you want to call it. I can be open, and they can be the same with me. As I am writing this, I am laughing, reminiscing about funny events with my friends and family. Do you ever take the time to hang out with friends, to text, e-mail, or chat about funny things? It's important to your health, and it's also important to your relationships.

Have you ever noticed the connection you have with people when you can laugh or share a joke? There is an emotional bonding experience for everyone involved; it's as though you're all on the same page.

When you laugh together, it helps keep a relationship new, silly, fresh, and definitely fun. When you laugh, it brings joy to everyone involved. It can also heal resentments, and it can definitely bring people closer together in difficult times. Incorporating laughter into your life can be a benefit to your children, your spouse, your family members, and your friends.

CREATING TIMES TO LAUGH

It's important to make laughter a part of your daily routine. Here are some ways to do so:

- Hang around with people who are funny and who like to laugh. I think I'm hysterical; what would your friends and family say about you?
- Watch a funny TV show or movie. I love sitting down with my family or friends when we can all laugh together.
- Goof around with your kids. Children are spontaneous and funny, and they're very honest with their feelings; in fact, children's laughter can be intoxicating. When my kids laugh, I close my eyes and just savor every sound.
- Play with your pet; animals also do some funny things.
- Go to a comedy club.

* Do something silly, such as playing jokes on people.
* Look for opportunities to just let go of your inhibitions.
* Make time to do fun activities.
* Smile.
* Write in your gratitude journal, as I talked about in the last chapter. When you are grateful and looking over your list, you will naturally feel happy, warm inside, and smiley.

A few years ago, my best friend Tammy and I went to see the awesome, motivating, and fun speaker Tony Robbins. Tony is one of the top transformational-leadership coaches in the world. He talked to us about laughter and how it changes the body's physiology. It helps our muscles, it helps our breathing, and it helps bring oxygen to our cells. If you've ever been to one of Tony's events, then you already know—you definitely laugh a lot. His events are filled with such positive energy; they're powerful and life-changing.

To me, life is about keeping things in perspective and not overreacting in situations, especially those we have zero control over. This is something you must keep on top of all the time. It's really a skill you can learn to develop and use when things are going wrong. Next time you're in a bad situation, try to laugh instead of succumbing to the negativity.

Life will bring about many challenges, especially when you are dealing with MS or any other health condition. I've learned there's value in taking a step back and making light of a situation; find some humor in it and then move on. I know you may say that this is easier said than done, but wouldn't you do anything to be healthier, more productive, and happier with your life? I know I would, and I continue to strive to have a better quality of life every day.

When you laugh, you open doors that you probably never knew existed, not only to your physical health, but also to your spiritual and mental health. You also open up the doors to creativity, to stronger relationships, to a more balanced lifestyle, and to a clearer vision of your future.

I know you may be thinking that some of the topics I'm discussing seem to be more about personal growth instead of health, but I tell you, they're all interconnected. You cannot be healthy if you are not whole in your mind, body, and spirit. That is one thing I've learned on this journey.

So, can we say laughter is the best medicine? Definitely!

CHAPTER 12
Juicing and Recipes

I JUICE ON A REGULAR basis. Because it's extremely healthy, I wanted to share this information. Juicing is an amazing way to strengthen our immune systems, and it's something the whole family can benefit from. I use an extracting juicer, which grinds up fruits and vegetables and then separates the pulp from the fruit. A blender mixes everything together, making more of a puree or smoothie. I use a juicer because my family prefers having less of a pulpy consistency to our drinks.

Fruits and vegetables contain vital nutrients that can help heal and restore our bodies, improve our gut health, and build up our immune systems. I fell in love with juicing for the mere fact that I can consume more fruits and vegetables in one sitting; all those essential nutrients are in one glass. When you juice daily, it helps your body flush out toxins. Juicing is essential to helping our cells. The big joke in my house is that when we are done juicing, our cells are singing. It sounds silly, but I believe it's the truth; your body just feels better after you drink some juice. It's interesting to see what happens to the body with a juicing program. You can lose weight, feel more energized, and actually stop craving all the fatty, sugary foods.

Health benefits of juicing:

* Juicing lowers your risk of heart disease

- Juicing strengthens your immune system
- Juicing regulates your metabolism
- Juicing energizes your body
- Juicing reduces your risk for chronic diseases and many types of cancers
- Juicing alkalizes and cleanses the body

Nutritionists and the USDA recommend eating five to nine servings of fresh fruits and vegetables each day. That seemed like a big number to me. I was always trying to find interesting ways to reach these goals for myself and my family. Juicing solves that challenge quite easily.

As I said in previous chapters, you are what you eat—your fruits and vegetables should be organic to ensure you're getting the best-quality nutrients without pesticides or other harmful chemicals. It's also important to forgo buying bottled juices, which may contain artificial colors, preservatives, and sweeteners.

The Environmental Working Group (EWG) has a great list of fruits and veggies that are safe to eat without being organic, and it also tells you the top chemical-laden fruits and veggies. The fruits and vegetables on the EWG's Dirty Dozen List tested positive for at least forty-seven different chemicals; others tested positive for up to sixty-seven. For produce on the EWG Dirty Dozen List, you should definitely go organic (unless, of course, you *want* to consume all those unhealthy, toxic chemicals). All the produce on the EWG Clean Fifteen List are least likely to have harmful pesticides or residues, and it is safe to consume nonorganic varieties. I recommend following the EWG on Facebook for the most up-to-date information on health or visiting their website, EWG.org.

The 2016 EWG Dirty Dozen List

* Strawberries
* Apples
* Nectarines
* Peaches
* Celery
* Grapes
* Cherries
* Spinach
* Tomatoes
* Sweet bell peppers
* Cherry tomatoes
* Cucumbers

The 2016 EWG Clean Fifteen List

* Avocados
* Corn (I only eat organic)
* Pineapples
* Cabbage
* Sweet peas (I only eat organic)
* Onions
* Asparagus
* Mangos
* Papayas (I only eat organic)
* Kiwis
* Eggplants
* Honeydew melons
* Grapefruit
* Cantaloupe
* Cauliflower

Some sweet corn, peas, and papayas are produced from genetically engineered seeds. Also GMO crops of papaya were introduced to Hawaii in the 1990s. So I also buy those organically, just to be safe.

Here are some of my favorite juicing recipes:

GREEN JUICE
1 Large Cucumber
1 Stalk of Celery
1 Handful of greens (kale or spinach)
1 or 2 Green or red apples
1 Sliver of ginger
1 Lemon (peeled)

GREEN JUICE 2
1 Large Cucumber
1 Stalk of Celery
4-5 Carrots
1 Sliver of ginger
1 Lemon (peeled)

GREEN JUICE 3
1 Cucumber
2 Handfuls of spinach
½ Beet
1 Stalk of celery
1 Sliver of ginger
2 Green apples

GREEN JUICE 4
2 Large cucumbers
3-4 Carrots
1 Handful of spinach
1 Stalk of celery
1 Handful of Cilantro
1 Sliver of ginger

CABBAGE JUICE
1 Half head of cabbage (Purple or Green)
3 Green apples
1 Sliver of ginger
4-5 Carrots

BEET TREAT
1 Large Beet
2 Cucumbers
1 Large sliver of ginger
1 Lime or lemon (peeled)

BEET TREAT 2
1 Large beet
1 Cucumber
1 Green or red apple
1 Sliver of ginger
2-3 Carrots

SUMMER 1
1 Lemon (peeled)
1 Pineapple (peeled)
1 Sliver of ginger
2-3 Green or red apples

FRUITY

2 Oranges (peeled)

2 Peaches (cut in half, remove seeds)

2-3 Green or red apples

1 Sliver of ginger

1-2 Handfuls blueberries, raspberries or blackberries

CARROTS

7-8 Carrots

3-4 Green or red apples

1 Sliver of ginger

DETOX GREEN

2 Cucumbers

2 Large handfuls of spinach

2 Stalks of celery

1 Handful of parsley

1 Handful of cilantro

1 Large sliver of ginger

REFRESH

2-3 Slices of watermelon

1 Lemon (peeled)

1 Sliver of ginger

2 Green or red apples

The great thing about juicing is that you can make up your own healthy concoctions. You may enjoy many other fruits, veggies, and herbs than I have listed. Another great thing about juicing is that you can't mess this up. You can also invite your kids to help you with this. It's a family-friendly project you all can enjoy!

CHAPTER 13

Conclusion

I HOPE YOU FOUND THIS book to be thought-provoking, helpful, motivating, and inspiring. Please know that this was a labor of love. I want everyone to truly know there is a better way to live. There is hope for all of us to have happy and productive lives while living with MS.

Yes, the road with MS can be paved with uncertainty, self-doubt, loneliness, and many challenges, but I hope you can incorporate some nuggets of information from this book every day.

Today, I still use a whole-home air-purification system. My family and I breathe clean, fresh air, day in and day out. I drink pH-balanced water to keep my body in an alkaline state. I clean my laundry with a technology that protects my health by giving me the ability to wash my clothes without detergents, fabric softeners, or bleaches. This protects my family from absorbing harmful, toxic chemicals into our skin—our largest organ. I take healthy, enzyme-based supplements, which had an immediate impact on my health when I started using them back in 2001 and continue to keep me strong every day. I drink a healthy, vitamin-packed energy drink that totally took away any signs of my chronic fatigue as well as my muscle aches and pains. (As I said in earlier chapters, I was taking two to three naps a day, which is no longer necessary.) I take an antioxidant-rich beverage that helps support circulation, immunity, nerve and brain function. Another great supplement I take is Liposomal C.

As MS sufferers, we need to look at healing our whole bodies rather than just treating our symptoms. If we want to be truly healthy, we need to look at what we breathe, what we eat, what we absorb, what our environments are, and even what relationships we choose to have. The green technologies and healthy supplements I discussed are amazing and have played a huge role in my transformation. I share about these products because all I can do is tell my story and talk about the things that I use consistently to transform my health.

I have learned so much throughout the years through education and investigation, and also by creating new partnerships and friendships with people who are very knowledgeable in healthy living.

In this whole process of healing, I've also learned that helping others is something I really enjoy, and it has led me to my purpose in life.

From my journey of waking up from MS, I've learned how to have a servant's attitude. I stopped worrying about my disease and started focusing on how I could start giving, whether it was through recommending healthy products, sharing information, or just offering friendship and support.

I have done many things to get where I am today. I am not giving medical advice; I am just sharing information about what is available to you and what I have personally done to heal *my* body and *beat* multiple sclerosis. Staying active, supplementing, utilizing green technologies, being positive, changing my diet, using holistic medicine, helping others, being grateful, and having good relationships has saved my life.

One thought I have to share about my journey is the fact that my pediatric neurologist was just awesome. He told me, "Kellie, don't worry about your MS; we will have a cure in five years!" So, being a kid, I believed him. Yes, I was naïve, but after I got over the initial shock of what MS was, that's how I lived my life. In my head, I always thought, *No worries; a cure is coming.* I never focused on MS. Remember, your mind-set is very important. I always *expected* a cure. I lived every day knowing and believing that a cure was coming. When you think about your life with MS, what are you expecting?

I want you to know that you have a choice about how you are going to live your life with MS. I often prayed that God would make me stronger. I prayed that God would put *good* people in my life to help me with my journey, and that is exactly what happened—and what continues to happen every day.

This year, 2017, is my twenty-ninth year of living with MS. I remember the early years as a struggle, being freaked out sometimes by some exacerbations and not understanding many things about this disease. We now live in the technology age, and we have so much vital information at our fingertips at any given moment. That being said, I also must caution you. Yes, we have so much information available to us, but that can also be a curse. If you're the type of person who goes online and looks up the worst-case scenarios about people and their MS, please stop doing that. If you're the type of person who immediately gets online to try to figure out every ache or pain, please stop doing that too. Our minds are far too powerful. The information you can find online will scare you, make you depressed, and take away your focus and your hope. Remember, what we think about, we bring about. My pediatric neurologist warned me not to read the info he gave my mom initially; he told me not to get caught up in the negative issues with this disease, as so many people will start to manifest the symptoms and conditions they read about.

The good news for all of us is that we now have many people paving the way for new ideas, new technologies, and new lives for those suffering from multiple sclerosis.

Start right now by writing out a detailed action plan of how you are going to fight this disease head-on. Remember, you have to be proactive with your health. I started this whole journey as if my MS was caused by a vitamin deficiency, and that was the foundation of my plan for healing.

Here are some of the things I did and continue to do to combat MS:

* I get a detailed blood panel of all my vitamin levels. (I do this two to four times a year, depending on my levels.)
* I analyze my vitamin-D intake—MS sufferers are chronically deficient in vitamin D; a blood test can tell you where you're at.
* I got tested for heavy metals.
* I examined my diet. I asked myself if what I was eating was unhealthy and what I could immediately add to my diet or take away that would benefit my health.
* I stopped using the microwave oven.
* I stay away from soda/pop. (I may have it once or twice a year, but generally, I try to avoid it.)
* I supplement daily with a whole-food, enzyme-packed multivitamin, probiotics, vitamin D-3 with K-2, a vitamin-packed energy drink, a functional beverage utilizing the muscadine grape, and Liposomal C.
* I became an avid label reader.
* Gluten-free
* I maintain an organic diet as much as possible.
* I am focused on ways to create the best body; I've listed many ways to do that and exactly how I used each of them (exercise,

massage, chiropractic care, acupuncture, meditation, journaling, and affirmations, etc.).

* I analyzed my relationships and evaluated how they were serving me. It's important to be around healthy-thinking people who support you and who've got your back.
* I lived in *hope* every day that I would beat this disease.

You have plenty of options and choices to start making these simple, healthy changes. It's time to get excited about your health and healing.

And remember my mantra: ***"A healthy immune system equals a healthy body!"***

I feel overjoyed, grateful, and blessed that I have been able to bring you my story. I pray this can be a stepping stone for you on your journey to *Waking Up from MS*. I look forward to sharing more information with you in other books, through my blog, *MS Free for ALL*, and on Facebook and Twitter. I cannot wait to hear about your own success story. *God Bless!*

I am not a physician. You should always follow the advice of your trusted health-care professional. I am sharing my personal experiences with you. This should not be substituted for medical advice.

REFERENCES

Chapter 1: My Story

Definition of RRMS - www.nationalmssociety.org

Chapter 2: What is MS?

Definition of MS - www.nationalmssociety.org

Chapter 3: MS Myths

Benefits of exercise - www.nationalmssociety.org

Chapter 4 – Just Say No

nationalmssociety.org/diseasemodifyingmedications
www.copaxone.com
www.tysabri.com
www.nationalmssociety.org/treating-MS/Novantrone
www.gilenya.com
www.tecfidera.com
www.aubagio.com

Chapter 5: Environmental Toxins

Smoking and MS – www.nationalmssociety.org/smoking
Lead In Your Water - www.usatoday.com
EWG's Guide to BPA - www.ewg.org/bpa
EWG's Guide to Safe Drinking Water - www.ewg.org/research/bottled-water-quality.

Chapter 7: You Are What You Eat

Overcoming Multiple Sclerosis Recovery Program - @georgejelinek. "Improving Life with Multiple Sclerosis | OvercomingMS." *Overcoming MS Homepage Comments.* N.p., n.d. Web. 08 Nov. 2016.

The Swank Diet - "Swank MS Foundation: For Your Health, For Your Future." *Swank MS Foundation.* N.p., n.d. Web. 08 Nov. 2016.

The Wahls Protocol - Wahls, Terry L., and Eve Adamson. *The Wahls Protocol: A Radical New Way to Treat all Chronic Autoimmune Conditions Using Paleo Principles.* New York: Avery, 2015. Print.

Campbell, T. Colin, and Thomas M.Campbell. *The China Study: The Most Comprehensive Study of Nutrition Ever Conducted and the Startling Implications for Diet, Weight Loss and Long-term Health.* Dallas, TX: BenBella, 2005. Print.

Schernhammer, E. S., K. A. Bertrand, B. M. Birmann, L. Sampson, W. C. Willett, and D. Feskanich. "Consumption of Artificial Sweetener- and Sugar-containing Soda and Risk of Lymphoma and Leukemia in Men and Women." *American Journal of Clinical Nutrition*96.6 (2012): 1419-428. Web.

Blaylock, Russell L. *Excitotoxins: The Taste That Kills.* Santa Fe, NM: Health, 1998. Print.

Chapter 8: Nutritional Supplementing

Vitamin D/evidence/dosing - mayoclinic.org/drugs-supplements/ vitamin-d/evidence.

Support for the Vitamin D Hypothesis for Multiple Sclerosis Risk." *Nature Clinical Practice Neurology* 3.7 (2007): 358. Web.

Fitzgerald, Susan. "A New Genetic Study Associates Low Vitamin D and Risk for Multiple Sclerosis." *Neurology Today* 15.18 (2015): 1. Web. UV Lights and Vitamin D - www.mercola.com.

Natarajan C, Bright JJ. Paper presented at the Annual Experimental Biology 2002 Conference New Orleans, LA April 23, 2002.

Chapter 9: Creating the best body

Sharma, Robin S. *The Monk Who Sold His Ferrari: A Fable about Fulfilling Your Dreams and Reaching Your Destiny*. Mumbai, India: Jaico Pub. House, 2006. Print.

Chapter 10: Give Me a Little More Attitude

Fredrickson, Barbara L. "What Good Are Positive Emotions?" *Review of General Psychology* 2.3 (1998): 300-19. Web.

Canfield, Jack, and Janet Switzer. *The Success Principles: How to Get from Where You Are to Where You Want to Be*. New York: Harper Resource Book, 2005. Print.

Chapter 11: Laughter

Roman, Lawrence, and Norman Cousins. *Anatomy of an Illness*. Los Angeles: Hamner/Gershwin Productions, 1982. Print

American College of Sports Medicine's 56th Annual Meeting in Seattle, 2009. (acsm.org/media-room/laugh-a-little-to-help-protect-heart-lower-blood-pressure)

20137204R00085

Made in the USA
San Bernardino, CA
26 December 2018